AIDS in an Aging Society
What We Need to Know

Matilda White Riley is Associate Director of Behavioral and Social Research, National Institute on Aging, National Institutes of Health and Professor Emerita of Sociology at Rutgers University and Bowdoin College. She is a member of the American Academy of Arts and Sciences and the Institute of Medicine (National Academy of Sciences). She has received an honorary L.H.D. and the Common Wealth Award in Sociology. Her publications include *Sociological Research* (two volumes), *Sociological Studies in Scale Analysis, Aging and Society* (three volumes), *Aging from Birth to Death* (two volumes), *Social Change and the Life Course* (two volumes), and numerous articles on mass communications, socialization, intergenerational relationships, research methods, and other topics.

Marcia G. Ory is Chief of Social Science Research on Aging, Behavioral and Social Research Program, National Institute on Aging, National Institutes of Health. She is very active in professional organizations and serves on several national task forces and advisory boards, including the Alzheimer's Disease and Related Disorders Association (ADRDA), Health Services Research Task Force, The Surgeon General's Workshop on Health Promotion and the Elderly, and the World Health Organization project on Health Behavior Research and Indicators. Dr. Ory's main interests and areas of research include aging, health, and behavior; aging and long-term care; gender differences in health and longevity; and implications of the AIDS epidemic for middle-aged and older populations.

Diane Zablotsky is a Social Science Analyst in the Behavioral and Social Research Program, National Institute on Aging, National Institutes of Health, and a doctoral candidate in Sociology at the University of Maryland, College Park. She has presented papers on family caregiving and is currently working on a dissertation investigating the relationship between older individuals' social support networks and their utilization of formal health care.

AIDS in an Aging Society

What We Need to Know

Matilda White Riley
Marcia G. Ory
Diane Zablotsky
Editors

Springer Publishing Company
New York

Springer Publishing Company, Inc.
536 Broadway
New York, NY 10012

89 90 91 92 93 / 5 4 3 2 1

Library of Congress Cataloging-in-Publication Data

AIDS in an aging society : what we need to know / edited by Matilda White Riley, Marcia G. Ory, Diane Zablotsky.
p. cm.
Includes bibliographies and index.
ISBN 0-8261-7060-9
1. AIDS (Disease)—United States. 2. AIDS (Disease)—Age factors. 3. Aged—Diseases. I. Riley, Matilda White, 1911- . II. Ory, Marcia G. III. Zablotsky, Diane.
[DNLM: 1. Acquired Immunodeficiency Syndrome—in old age. WD 308 A2883383]
RA644.A25A36353 1989
618.97'69792—dc19
DNLM/DLC
for Library of Congress 89-5863
CIP

Printed in the United States of America

CONTENTS

Part III Care

Part IV Societal Consequences

PREFACE

We know that AIDS (acquired immune deficiency syndrome) is an epidemic that involves not only young adults but also middle-aged and older people. We know too that behavior and life-style are major factors in preventing the disease, in transmitting it, and in coping with the burden of care. Yet the social and behavioral sciences have as yet provided little systematic knowledge about *how* older people are involved in the epidemic, or about *what* can be done to reduce the threats posed by this dreaded disease to the increasing number of older people within the United States population as a whole.

NEED FOR THE BOOK

Deeper understanding of AIDS in an aging society is needed for many reasons. Perhaps first among them is that the risks for spread of the AIDS epidemic, and the potential for controlling it, cannot be fully assessed without much further information about the sexual activity and the vulnerability to HIV infection of the large and growing number of people beyond the reproductive ages. Second, in view of the uniquely fatal, infectious, and currently stigmatized character of AIDS, new knowledge is needed about the behavior changes and prevention strategies that could minimize transmission of AIDS among older individuals. Third, the health care of older people, already a crisis in many parts of the country, will certainly be affected by the competing demands of an AIDS epidemic. Yet little information is at hand as to the extent of these competing demands or to reactions by frail older people to claimants for care who are suffering from AIDS. (One example points to a tendency to resist sharing the long-term care system: It is reported that no nursing homes in New York City are willing to accept AIDS patients—*New York Times,* October 13, 1988.) Even within families, who are far more important than institutions as providers of care, it is not known how older people, who grew up prior to the "sexual revolution," will respond when relatives with AIDS come home to them to be cared for.

On these counts and many others, detailed examination of the knowledge already available in the social and behavioral sciences is required in order to deal effectively with AIDS among people in later life. Even more importantly, dealing with the AIDS epidemic before it is too late to control its spread requires identification of areas where essential new knowledge ought to be obtained.

PURPOSE AND AUDIENCE

This book aims to address these needs. Its chapters illustrate what we are beginning to know and indicate what we still need to know about the social and behavioral implications of AIDS among middle-aged and older people. Thus the book speaks to social scientists, students of the life course and the aging society, and scholars in the many disciplines concerned with HIV and AIDS and their far-reaching implications. The book also speaks to those in professional practice and public policy, who can utilize the emerging knowledge base as a guide in designing appropriate, timely, and critically needed interventions. And it offers information, as well as cautions, for people of all ages, who, if not afflicted themselves, will predictably confront persons with AIDS in their families or communities. In particular, this book challenges researchers who can help to fill gaps in the rapidly accumulating body of knowledge.

BACKGROUND OF THE BOOK

The book grew out of work initiated in 1987 by the Behavioral and Social Research Program of the National Institute on Aging (NIA), National Institutes of Health. At that time, we became aware of the general neglect, in the expanding research on AIDS, of the implications for older people—despite the late-life vulnerability to disease, and despite the fact that in many families older people are becoming the givers, rather than the receivers, of care. At that time, too, we became aware of the special responsibilities imposed on us at NIA by the overriding role of social and behavioral factors, not only in transmission of the virus, but also in preventing or coping with the disease. As the then Secretary of Health and Human Services, Otis Bowen, put it, the problem of AIDS is primarily a problem of *behavior*.

Having determined that we should develop a program for funding research grants on AIDS, we considered how to alert scientists in the many relevant fields to the challenges, opportunities, and problems in this area. As one approach, we commissioned a number of state-of-the-art papers from experts with varied backgrounds. The papers addressed selected portions of the general topic, *Social and Behavioral Aspects of AIDS in the Middle and Later Years.*

To discuss these papers, NIA held a Workshop on AIDS in May 1988, aiming to assess the existing knowledge and identify missing links in this knowledge. The authors of the papers, who led the discussions, were joined by others working on AIDS from other agencies and with different perspectives (including the National Institute of Child Health and Human Development, the National Institute of Mental Health, the Centers for Disease Control, the National Center for Health Services Research, the National Center for Health Statistics, the National Academy of Sciences, the Office of the Surgeon General, etc.). The wide participation in the deliberations, and the consensual enthusiasm that developed, are indicative of the strong collaborative basis for pursuing this initiative.

Many of these papers now constitute the substance of the present volume.[1] They have been revised by the authors and supplemented by newly added papers. Moreover, they have been extensively edited, partly to give coherence to the volume as a whole and partly to avoid excessive repetition—although repetition of certain key points in different contexts often adds to the meaning of the point, as well as serving to emphasize it.

ACKNOWLEDGMENTS

Advice, scientific guidance, and moral and financial support for this project have been provided by numerous colleagues. Within the National Institute on Aging these include the members of the NIA AIDS Coordinating Committee: William Adler, Andrea LaCroix, Andrew Monjan, Huber Warner, and most particularly Samuel Korper. Within sister institutes and agencies these colleagues include all those attending the NIA workshop, with special recognition to William Darrow of the Centers for Disease Control and to Duane Alexander and Wendy Baldwin from the National Institute for Child Health and Human Development. To all these persons and agencies the editors express deep appreciation. Their final indebtedness is to John W. Riley, Jr., who supplied unstinting editorial advice and criticism throughout the preparation of this book.

M.W.R., M.G.O., D.Z.

[1] Despite NIA's involvement in stimulating the papers and in editing them, however, it must be made clear that the facts and opinions stated are entirely the responsibility of the respective authors, and do not necessarily reflect official positions either of NIA or of the editors.

CONTRIBUTORS

Gary L. Albrecht is a Professor at the University of Illinois School of Public Health. He is editor of *The Sociological Quarterly* and Chair of the Medical Sociology Section of the American Sociological Association. He has published extensively in the sociology of health and juvenile justice arenas. His present research focuses on the methodological problems of conducting research on sensitive issues in the general population, the effect of fear of AIDS on behavior, and AIDS as a chronic disease.

Joseph A. Catania is a Research Psychologist with the Division of General Internal Medicine and Senior Scientist with the Center for AIDS Prevention Studies at the University of California, San Francisco. He is the author of numerous articles in the areas of sexuality and aging, sexuality research methods, and primary prevention aspects of AIDS. He is currently conducting research on the determinants of high-risk sexual behavior and condom use among heterosexual and gay adults and adolescents.

Thomas J. Coates is Associate Professor of Medicine, Director of the Behavioral Medicine Unit, and Co-Director of the Center for AIDS Prevention Studies (CAPS) at the University of California, San Francisco. He has done extensive research in health behavior change, particularly in the area of smoking cessation and hypertension management. Since 1983, he has been involved in AIDS research, focusing especially on strategies for reducing the spread of infection.

Stephen Crystal is Chair, Division on Aging, Director, AIDS Research Group, and Associate Research Professor at the Institute for Health, Health Care Policy, and Aging Research, Rutgers University. He is the author of *America's Old Age Crises: Public Policy and the Two Worlds of Aging,* senior author of *The Management of Home Care Services* (Springer, 1987), and recipient of the Abt Associates Prize in Public Policy Research. He writes on a range of issues both in AIDS and aging policy and is currently principal investigator for several AIDS policy studies and for research on the economics of aging. Dr. Crystal's longstanding involvement with long-term care policy has included numerous evaluations and policy studies (including current evaluation of New Jersey's Medicaid waiver program for AIDS care). His research has included studies of health services utilization and psychosocial adaptation of persons with AIDS in San Diego and in New Jersey.

Yasmine Ergas is a Staff Associate at the Social Science Research Council, New York City. She spent 1987–88 on leave from the Council as a member of the Institute for Advanced Study (Princeton, New Jersey). She has published extensively on gender politics, public policies, and social movements, and has worked on the use of autobiographical documents and life narratives in the social sciences and the humanities.

Susan M. Kegeles is a Research Psychologist with the Division of General Internal Medicine and Senior Scientist with the Center for AIDS Prevention Studies at the University of California, San Francisco. She is the author of numerous articles on adolescent risk-taking behavior and adult and adolescent contraceptive decision-making. She is currently conducting research on the antecedent of AIDS risk behavior and is developing interventions to reduce risky behavior.

Judith A. Levy is Assistant Professor of Health Resources Management, School of Public Health, University of Illinois at Chicago. Dr. Levy is active in numerous professional organizations and currently serves as President of the Midwest Council for Social Research on Aging. She is co-editing a book on disability across the life course and another on health care occupations. She has published in the areas of aging and health, the sociology of death and dying, and social movements in medicine. Her most recent work focuses on the knowledge, attitudes, and behavior of the general population toward AIDS.

G. David Maddox is a Research Biologist for the Maryland Natural Heritage Program. He has published many papers on population biology, genetics, and evolution. His current research concerns the biology of endangered species.

George L. Maddox is Professor of Sociology and of Medical Sociology (Psychiatry) and Chairman of the Council on Aging and Human Development at Duke University. He directed Duke's multidisciplinary Center on Aging and Human Development from 1972 to 1982. He is editor-in-chief of the *Encyclopedia of Aging* and is author or editor of a number of recent books and articles on epidemiological and socioeconomic aspects of adult development and aging. He is the recipient of the Sandoz International Prize for Research on Aging, the Kleemeier Research Award of the Gerontological Society of America, and the Distinguished Contribution to Aging Award of the American Sociological Association and is a Fellow of the American Association for the Advancement of Science.

John B. McKinlay is Vice-President and Director of the New England Research Institute, a private research organization specializing in epidemiology, gerontology, health services research, and social policy. He is also Professor of Sociology and Research Professor of Medicine at Boston University and holds appointments at the Beth Israel and Massachusetts General Hospitals (Harvard Medical School). He is editor, author, and co-author of numerous books and professional papers, and a consultant to national governments, state agencies, and international organizations on matters of health and social policy issues. In 1987 he received the MERIT Award from the National Institute on Aging.

Kenneth G. Manton is Research Professor of Demographic Studies at Duke University and Medical Research Professor at Duke University Medical Center's Department of Community and Family Medicine. Dr. Manton is also a Senior Fellow of the Duke University Medical Center's Center for the Study of Aging and Human Development and Assistant Director of the Duke University Center for Demographic Studies. In 1986 he was named head of the World Health Organization Collaborating Center for Research and Training in the Methods of Assessing Risk and Forecasting Health Status Trends as Related to Multiple Disease Outcomes, based at the Center for Demographic Studies. His current research interests include forecasting morbidity, disability, and mortality among the nation's elderly, reimbursement maintenance of quality of care for both acute and long-term care services consumed by the elderly, mathematical modeling at advanced ages, and differentials in those processes by sex and race and cross-nationally. He has published extensively in these areas, including a forthcoming book with Eric Stallard, *Chronic Disease Modelling: Measurement and Evaluation of the Risk of Chronic Disease Processes.*

Lance Pollack is the database manager for the Psychological Division of the Center for AIDS Prevention Policy at the University of California, San Francisco, as well as a doctoral candidate in the Human Development and Aging Program at the same university. He is currently working on a dissertation concerning the sociological aspects of the retirement transition.

John W. Riley, Jr., Consulting Sociologist, has had two major careers. After teaching for some 30 years, he became a senior officer at The Equitable, where he was in charge of corporate affairs, including health. He has served as President of the Sociological Research Association and the American Association for Public Opinion Research, from which he received the Distinguished

Award in 1983. In 1987 the American Sociological Association gave him the Distinguished Career Award for the Practice of Sociology, and he is the recipient of an honorary L.L.D. In recent years he has played an active role in several major projects on health promotion and self-care. Over the years he has specialized in studies of dying and the meaning of death.

Burton Singer is Professor of Biostatistics and Public Health, Economics, and Statistics at Yale University and Professor at Rockefeller University. His outstanding leadership in mathematical modeling and applied statistics is reflected in his numerous publications and professional presentations. Formerly Co-Chair of the Advisory Board for the Columbia University Center for Applied Social Research, he chairs the Committee on Statistics of the National Academy of Sciences. Among his many honors, he is a Fellow of the American Association for the Advancement of Science.

Katherine Skinner has a strong surgical and gerontological nursing background. Her current research interest focuses on the interface between formal and informal caregiving of the elderly. Other areas of interest include the health of women veterans and health care utilization among the elderly. Her most recent work examines the relevance and application of social science perspectives as the AIDS epidemic spreads among the elderly.

Sherry E. Spitzer is currently the Project Director for the Transfusion Notification Program at Children's Hospital, Oakland. She is also a Research Associate at the University of California, San Francisco (UCSF) Center for AIDS Prevention Studies, and works with the San Francisco AIDS Foundation. Although Dr. Spitzer's major focus and most recent publications concern AIDS-related topics, other strong research interests include cognitive and educational applications of visual and verbal thinking.

Ron Stall is an Assistant Adjunct Professor in the Epidemiology and International Health Department at the University of California, San Francisco and a senior scientist at the Center for AIDS Prevention Studies at the same institution. His primary research interests have centered on the study of alcohol-related behaviors across the life course, in particular among the elderly. He has also written a series of papers concerning the prevention of HIV infection. These have primarily centered on the identification of the circumstances under which individuals decline to comply with health education messages concerning the prevention of HIV infection. Currently Dr. Stall is the principal investigator of a study that seeks to develop a model of care for intravenous drug users with AIDS, is a study director for a World Health Organization study of AIDS risk reduction among gay and bisexual men being conducted in 12 countries, and is engaged in the continuing analysis of a set of longitudinal AIDS data being conducted in San Francisco.

Heather Turner is a doctoral student in the Human Development and Aging Program and Research Assistant at the Center for AIDS Prevention Studies (CAPS) at the University of California, San Francisco. Her research interests involve the psychosocial factors relating to mental health. Her most recent work has focused on the sources and mediators of stress among AIDS caregivers and issues surrounding the risk of AIDS for older people.

PART I

Introduction

CHAPTER 1

AIDS and Older People: The Overlooked Segment of the Population

Matilda White Riley

Everyone knows that we live in an aging society. Over one quarter of the population is aged 50 and over, about one-eighth are 65 and over, and the number of people in these age categories is continually rising. And we know a great deal about these older people—their characteristics and their problems. What *no* one knows—and what few have even considered—is how AIDS is affecting these millions of middle-aged and older people.[1] This oversight is based on widespread assumptions that are largely false. It is often assumed that beyond young adulthood AIDS prevention efforts would be wasted. Some even assume that sexual activity stops in mid-life. The facts are, however, that 10% of the AIDS cases that have been diagnosed in the United States have occurred among people aged 50 and over, including 1% who had reached or passed age 65. According to the 1988 reports, that 1% represents 1,000 older people with AIDS. And, intolerable as it seems, these numbers are steadily increasing and appear likely to explode in the near future as those already infected, who are growing older year by year, develop AIDS or AIDS-related illnesses.

As a sociologist unschooled in the biomedical sciences, though fully impressed with the important interactions between biomedical and psychosocial processes affecting both AIDS and aging, I embark upon this chapter with considerable temerity. In addition to the dedicated assistance of my co-editors (they too are sociologists), I am especially indebted for expert advice and criticism on earlier versions of this chapter to Joshua Lederberg and Zeda Rosenberg, and also to Lois Cohen, John Kalberer, Dushanka Kleinman, and Andrew Monjan. Jeannette Perry and Virginia Morgan were helpful in manuscript preparation. The responsibility for erroneous or misleading statements is, of course, entirely my own.

[1] As late as 1986, the index to a wide-ranging collection of essays on *Our Aging Society* (Pifer and Bronte) contains not a single reference to the topic of AIDS.

This book is about AIDS in this overlooked segment of the population. Among children, as well as among women and minorities, special efforts toward research and prevention are already under way. Meanwhile, however, the special vulnerabilities of older people are generally neglected. We want to emphasize at the outset two of the most serious implications of this oversight:

- First, the large and rapidly growing number of people in the middle-aged and older segment of the United States population may well constitute the last major frontier for prevention of AIDS. This presents an early opportunity to begin prevention efforts now, to forestall any possibility that the epidemic may become strongly entrenched among the more than 60 million people aged 50 and over. Here is an opportunity to learn from previous failures with the populations first afflicted with AIDS: homosexual and bisexual males, intravenous drug abusers, and their sexual partners, any one of whom may unwittingly already be infected.
- Second, the head-on competition for long-term care between frail older people and people with AIDS is exacerbating the already heavy care burdens on families, communities, and society as a whole. A great deal is known about the problems of caring for older people, currently the major users of long-term care, and about potential means of helping to alleviate the burdens of care. Here is an opportunity to learn from the experience with the frail elderly, before the emerging demands for care of AIDS patients reach crisis proportions.

We believe that these two considerations—among many others—present a unique and immediate challenge to take advantage of these opportunities to prevent further spread of AIDS and to confront the problems of long-term care. Both these opportunities require immediate interventions that are social and behavioral, while the biomedical sciences seek vaccines, treatments, and cures. In the future, as medical science advances, the principles, knowledge, and research skills of the social and behavioral sciences will continue to be needed—in implementing new medical knowledge, in coping with the social implications, and in contributing to basic understanding of the societal course and consequences of this and possible future epidemics. The chapters in this book address this challenge.

The first section of this introductory chapter describes the rapidly changing background of these discussions, as new knowledge and emerging patterns of the disease complicate our efforts to examine what we need to know about AIDS (Acquired Immune Deficiency Syndrome). The second section then turns to the relationship of age to AIDS, showing how age serves as a mediator between disease outcomes and a variety of social, cultural, and psychological factors. It also shows how the prolonged natural history of the disease coincides with the processes of growing older and can be examined in the light of existing knowledge of these processes. The third section describes the major purposes of each of the diverse chapters and shows how these chapters are located in the three parts of the book, which emphasize respectively risk factors and prevention, care, and societal consequences. Supplementing and integrating the contributions of these chapters, Part IV of the book identifies several conceptual and methodological strands from the social and behavioral sciences that can be utilized in our search for understanding AIDS in an aging society. Thus this search need not start entirely from scratch.

THE SHIFTING SCENE: A CAUTIONARY NOTE

Before any attempt is made to address the opportunities for prevention and for coping with care, a strong emphasis on caution is in order. The situation is continually changing, often in unexpected ways. Hence the caveat: *Whatever can be said about AIDS today* (apart from the ways in which it is spread) *is likely to be untrue tomorrow.* Current reports are often inaccurate—based on biased samples and incomplete data (e.g., the official United States surveillance reports are said to cover only some 80% or 90% of the AIDS cases—inaccuracies that are discussed in several chapters in this volume). Thus, as knowledge accumulates and becomes more nearly accurate, the reports change.[2] Even more important than shifting reports of the facts are alterations in the facts themselves, for both the patterns of the disease and the surrounding social environment are continually in flux. All these types of changes must be kept in mind in reading this book and in working with the issues it raises. Just a few examples are described here at the outset.

Changes and Variabilities in Definitions of the Disease

One major shift that has occurred involves the scientific definitions of the nature of the disease and the criteria used in diagnosis. In 1982, the official definition used by the Centers for Disease Control (CDC) required the presence of malignancies and certain "opportunistic infections" (i.e., infections that occur because the immune function has broken down [Redfield & Burke, 1988]); in August 1987, the CDC revised this definition to include

[2] Many statements in this chapter rely on recent reports, still in preparation at the time of writing, including that of the National Academy of Sciences Committee for the Oversight of AIDS Activities (Turner, Miller, and Moses, 1989); and the Charlottesville report of the Second AIDS Prevention and Control Meeting, U.S. Public Health Service (forthcoming in *Public Health Reports,* 1988).

dementia and wasting syndrome. In 1988, the earlier distinction between those who "have" or "do not have" AIDS was being changed to the notion of HIV infection as a "continuum of conditions associated with immune dysfunction." Rather than speaking only of AIDS as the disease, it has been suggested that perhaps the HIV infection itself should be considered the disease. HIV, or the human immunodeficiency virus, is now known to cause, as Redfield and Burke (p. 90) put it, "a predictable, progressive derangement of the immune system," of which "AIDS is just one, late manifestation."

Further confounding the complexity of these definitional changes are variabilities observed when the United States is compared with other parts of the world. Whereas in the United States the majority of cases have so far occurred among homosexual and bisexual males and urban IV drug abusers, in most of Africa and parts of the Caribbean most cases occur among heterosexuals. In one United States city, New York, AIDS is reported as the leading cause of death for men aged 25 to 44 and for women aged 25 to 34, whereas a report from Kinshasha, Zaire, a city with one of the highest HIV infection rates in the world, cites AIDS as the cause of 26% of all deaths of people between the ages of 15 and 20 (*New York Times,* 10/10/88). Not only do patterns of disease vary from one country to another, but different forms of the virus are observed (e.g., HIV-2 rather than HIV-1). In the meantime the virus itself is changing in unpredictable ways as mutations occur.[3]

Clearly, such changes and variabilities in the disease and in its definitions pose major difficulties in interpreting the discussions in this book. They affect the very phenomena for which epidemiological trends are being plotted; for example, the 1988 reports of surveillance data on older people (to be presented in this chapter) cannot readily be compared directly with data for the earlier years (presented in subsequent chapters). Moreover, revisions in definition will predictably influence the very public health measures and clinical treatments that are being examined here as implicating the older population.

Changes in the Subpopulations of Concern

When AIDS first moved into the United States in the late 1970s (in 1977, as reported by Dawson, 1988), it took on a special character. Introduced into large metropolitan areas among male homosexuals and bisexuals and abusers of intravenous drugs, it became entrenched in these enclaves before widespread prevention efforts were initiated. More recently, scientific and professional attention has been turned to the vulnerabilities among heterosexual

[3] This type of virus is particularly subject to mutations, which can occur even within a single person as host (personal conversation with Joshua Lederberg, 10/21/88). There is much debate about whether possible mutations are sufficient to prevent detection by current diagnostic tests, but the hope is that these tests can be assumed to be adequate.

women as well as men; among minority populations; and among the children of mothers infected with the virus (HIV).[4]

Meanwhile, as emphasized in the title of this chapter, it is the older people who continue to elude attention. As one small example, a *New York Times* report (10/7/88) of a CDC investigation of the 1986 rise in city deaths from pneumonia cites AIDS as a possible concomitant, but the report focused only on males aged 25 to 44—in spite of the fact that most pneumonia-associated deaths occur among older people, where AIDS might also be implicated. That blood transfusions are common among older people is recognized; but concern for this source of AIDS transmission was reduced (though continued spread of the virus was not eliminated) by introduction in 1985 of screening of blood and blood products for use in transfusion. Less well recognized is the fact that unprotected homosexual and bisexual practices constitute the primary transmission sources for people over, as well as under, age 50 (see Chapter 5 by Catania and others)—though the extent of these practices at any age is not known. In most serious research, including the research funded by major federal programs, the neglect of the older population is conspicuous.

However, there is still time to overcome this neglect before the epidemic is allowed to spread widely within this last frontier of men and women in the middle and later years.

Changes in Public Attitudes and Knowledge about AIDS

Associated with the changes in the subpopulations involved in the epidemic are gradual shifts in the way AIDS is viewed, as well as small increments in public awareness of what is happening. AIDS may become less stigmatized if the spreading epidemic becomes less closely identified with the opprobrium attached to gays, bisexual males, and drug abusers. As one example of the changing cultural landscape, in October 1988 the U.S. Justice Department, reversing its 1986 ruling, prohibited discrimination against persons with AIDS in employment and in programs receiving federal funds (*Washington Post,* 10/7/88). Education, increasing public awareness, and familiarity with others who have the disease are helping the public to draw the narrow line between appropriate measures of prevention and unwarranted fears of infection from casual contact.[5]

All such changes in public attitudes and knowledge come slowly at every age, however, and there are indications that they come most slowly of all

[4] See, e.g., the cross-cutting topics for federally funded research, as noted in the Charlottesville report.

[5] Although no example of airborne transmission of HIV has been documented, Joshua Lederberg (1988b) cautions that AIDS patients with tuberculosis and terminal pneumonia are another potential hazard. In view of the grave consequences of pneumonic dissemination, should it occur, he cautions that more research is urgently needed on the emission of HIV accompanying such disease.

among older people (Dawson, 1988). People 50 and over, when compared in a cross-sectional survey with younger people, are less aware of the risks of getting the AIDS virus: as of mid-1988, 84% of those 50 and over, as compared with 65% of those aged 18 to 29, thought they had *no* chance of getting the virus. Older people are comparatively less likely to have been tested for HIV-specific antibodies (frequently and erroneously referred to as the "AIDS blood test"), or to be willing to be tested. They are less likely to have discussed AIDS with relatives or friends, and less certain that a person who has AIDS can look healthy and well. They are somewhat less knowledgeable about how HIV infection does occur (through sexual contact with an infected person, injection with infected blood, or perinatal transmission); and they are also less sure about how infection does *not* occur (by using public toilets, sharing plates and glasses, or shaking hands with an infected person). (For details, see Chapter 3 by Levy & Albrecht in this volume; also American Public Health Association, 1988.)

As knowledge and attitudes about AIDS change, the changes can enhance the effectiveness of public education and other efforts toward prevention. Moreover, increases in knowledge and in motivation to protect against the disease could certainly affect behaviors and life-styles of both the infected and noninfected, and these increases could also influence the care given to people with AIDS, and thus potentially the course of the disease. Nevertheless, there is a long step between knowledge and behavior change. In Kinshasha, Zaire, where awareness of AIDS is almost universal, over half feel they themselves are at no risk—"AIDS happens to other people, not to me" (*New York Times,* October 10, 1988).

In sum, this book describes a continually shifting scene. The nature of AIDS, the populations it attacks, the public views toward it, and the virus itself are all in flux. In the meantime, the society is aging: Increasing numbers of people in the United States are middle-aged or old. Moreover, all these changes are interactive: Each continually influences the others. And they complicate the diverse attempts throughout this book to examine what we believe we already know, and what we still need to know.

RELATION BETWEEN AGE AND AIDS

As the scene shifts and as increasingly accurate information about the nature and epidemiology of AIDS and HIV is accumulating, the relationships of AIDS to the aging society and to the individual aging processes is becoming increasingly complex. The epidemic is taking such diverse symptomatic and asymptomatic forms that it is now often called an HIV epidemic rather than an AIDS epidemic. Increasingly it threatens—either directly or indirectly—all segments of the society, including the large numbers of middle-aged and older people. And for the afflicted individual, the long natural history of the disease, from infection to full-blown AIDS, interacts in varied ways with the biopsychosocial processes of aging.

Age Patterns of the AIDS Epidemic

AIDS in the United States is generally regarded as a young persons' disease, striking most heavily those in the productive years. Nevertheless, this book postulates (1) that middle-aged and older people also are affected, both actually and potentially; and (2) that age, rather than being a cutoff point, acts as a mediator between many significant social, cultural, and behavioral factors and the disease outcomes.

As true indicators of the still uncharted spread of the disease, data are needed, not so much on clinical cases of AIDS as on the epidemiology of the HIV virus. Unfortunately, however, few data are available on the numbers with evidence of prior infection (HIV-antibody positive), save for rough estimates of one to one-and-a-half million persons in the United States (Heyward & Curran, 1988), or of 5 to 10 million worldwide (Mann et al., 1988). Moreover, there are no systematic reports of age patterns of these infected persons, many of whom are unaware that they are infected. What is known is that their numbers are so large as to warrant the hackneyed metaphor that, at every age, the diagnosed AIDS cases constitute only the tip of the proverbial iceberg.[6]

At present, the best available statistics for the United States derive not from the cases of HIV infection but from the cases diagnosed as having AIDS as these are reported to the Centers for Disease Control (CDC) and accumulated in the CDC Weekly Surveillance Reports. These data expunge any misconception that AIDS is confined to young people. Instead, there is a considerable scattering across the full age range, as shown in Table 1.1. This table presents the age distribution of the approximately 73,000 cases of AIDS that had been reported to the CDC from 1981 up to August, 1988.[7] To be sure, nearly half of these cases (46%) were people in their thirties. However, another 21% were in their forties, while 10% were aged 50 and over. In short, with use of chronological age as a

[6] Worthy of investigation is the question of whether the ratio of AIDS prevalence to HIV prevalence may be somewhat smaller among older than among younger people, as death rates in general tend to increase at the oldest ages, or as blood transfusions—which can deliver massive infusions of the virus—are widespread among older people.

[7] It must be emphasized that these figures are not incidence or prevalence rates, since the denominators or bases for the percentages are not available. Moreover, while new cases are being reported, their accumulating numbers are being steadily winnowed by death: by September, 1988, 56% of the 73,000 reported cases had died (Centers for Disease Control, 1987, *Weekly Surveillance Report*).

TABLE 1.1 Age Distribution of AIDS Cases Reported in the United States Pre-1981 to September, 1988

Age	Number	Percent
Under 5	977	1
5–12	194	*
13–19	295	*
20–29	15,163	21
30–39	33,951	46
40–49	15,287	21
Over 49	7,527	10
Total cases	73,394[a]	100

* = less than 1%

[a]Includes 9,720 patients who meet only the 1987 revised surveillance definition for AIDS; thus not directly comparable with data for earlier years.

Note: Of the 73,394 cases, 41,393 (56%) are known to have died.

Source: Centers for Disease Control (CDC) Weekly Surveillance Reports—cumulative totals

crude marker, nearly one third of the cases diagnosed with AIDS have already passed early adulthood.

Old Age

Further detail on new cases of older people with AIDS, as contrasted with the total AIDS cases at all ages, is shown in Table 1.2 (the data for which were specially prepared by the CDC for this book). Of the over 7,000 people aged 50 or over diagnosed with AIDS (bottom row of the table), 1,000 had reached or passed age 65—a number even greater than the number (977) of babies and children under age 5 with AIDS. These findings further demonstrate the wide age range of the epidemic.

Modes of Transmission

Table 1.2 also shows the percentage distributions of these cases according to the primary[8] modes of transmission of AIDS. Of considerable interest is the similarity between those aged 50 to 64 (column 1) and the total for all ages

[8] Certain artifacts of this classification may be especially relevant for the older population, since cases with more than one risk factor are tabulated only in the category listed first (*AIDS Weekly Surveillance Reports*). Thus, for example, a homosexual male with AIDS would be so classified and would not be counted again under "transfusions"—even if he were in fact infected from the latter source.

TABLE 1.2 AIDS Cases in the United States, Older People and All Ages (Percent Distribution by Age and Transmission Category)

	Age 50+[a]			
Transmission category	50–64 %	65+ %	Total 50+ %	All Ages[b] %
Homosexual/bisexual male	68	26	62	63
Intravenous (IV) drug user	10	2	8	19
Homosexual male & IV drug user	2	1	2	7
(Total homosexual/bisexual)	(70)	(27)	(64)	(70)
(Total IV drug user)	(12)	(3)	(10)	(26)
Hemophilia	1	4	2	1
Heterosexual cases	3	4	3	4
Transfusion, blood components	9	55	16	3
Undetermined	7	8	7	3
Total cases = 100%	6,167	1,008	7,175	72,223

[a] Pre-1981 to August, 1988

[b] Pre-1981 to September, 1988. Excludes children under 13.

Source: Centers for Disease Control (CDC) Weekly Surveillance Reports—cumulative totals.

(column 4). For both, homosexual and bisexual males constitute the primary source of transmission (70%). Intravenous (IV) drug abusers, though they rank second (12%) as the source for people 50–64, are considerably less important for those ages than for the total (26%).

Markedly different from the younger categories are those people with AIDS who are aged 65 and over (column 3). For them the largest source is blood transfusion (55%); though, even here, homosexual and bisexual males are also significant (27%).

Race and Sex

Two other distinguishing characteristics of AIDS cases generally—race and sex—are important descriptors also of cases occurring at the later ages (data supplied by CDC, not shown here). By race, 42% of the total cases consist of minorities (primarily blacks and Hispanics), in contrast to some 20% in the United States population. At older ages, a similar but less pronounced pattern of AIDS appears: 33% of those aged 50 to 64 are minorities, and 19% of those 65 and over.

By sex, the striking phenomenon (compatible with the predominance of male homosexuality and bisexuality as a source of transmission) is that 91% of the total cases have been male, only 9% female. In both of the older age categories, male cases still predominate, constituting 94% of those aged 50 to 64 and 76% of those 65 and over. In both older age categories, the male cases were proportionately more likely than the female to have contracted the disease from male homosexuals or bisexuals, whereas the female cases were proportionately more likely to have arisen from blood transfusion or heterosexual contact. Among the female AIDS cases aged 50 to 64, of which there were 376, heterosexual contact accounted for as many as 27%, with another 41% traced to transfusion. (As expected, transfusion was proportionately still higher—78%—for female cases aged 65 and over.)

These patterns of transmission are difficult to interpret, since they represent percentage distributions of AIDS cases rather than rates of prevalence or incidence. Nevertheless, these patterns raise critical questions for the future. How far will the epidemic spread among older people within the minority populations? And as AIDS among younger people reaches farther beyond the minorities into the majority white population, will older whites also become increasingly affected? Perhaps even more critical is the potential for heterosexual transmission to females, including older women. Are the existing sex differentials entirely matters of cultural diffusion? Or are there biological differences between the sexes in vulnerability to AIDS?

Trends

The picture of the AIDS cases reported during the 1980s is anything but static, as shown in detail by Stall and his associates in Chapter 4 of this volume. (See Tables 4.1 and 4.4.) To be sure, the age distribution has remained remarkably stable since the inception (beginning with the pre-1981 years) of the CDC Weekly Surveillance Reports: approximately 10% of the cases have occurred among people 50 and over. Yet in every age category the number of cases has been increasing. And from year to year there have been small but consistent changes in the relative importance of the sources of transmission. In most age categories (those aged 20–29 are the exception), homosexual and bisexual males, still the overwhelmingly predominant source of infection, have nevertheless become comparatively less important, whereas the proportion of cases traceable to IV drug abuse has been increasing. These general trends apply also to those aged 50 and over, where there are similar increases in the proportions emanating from both transfusion and heterosexual contact.

For the future, of course, it is the hidden epidemic of HIV infection that is critical. For example, one estimate postulates that, after taking account of increasing rates of infection, there may be as many as 365,000 cases of full-blown AIDS in the United States by 1992 (Heyward & Curran, 1988).[9] Every infected

[9] For discussion of information about HIV required for more accurate forecasts of future numbers of AIDS cases, see Chapters 4 (by Stall, Catania, and Pollack) and 9 (by Manton and Singer) in this volume.

person is continually growing older and thus—up until death or the discovery of a cure—potentially contributing to the future pool of older people with AIDS.

In summary, then, the situation of older people with AIDS today may well foreshadow future patterns in the United States as a whole. In the current scene, older people are seen to reflect the general patterns of AIDS among people of all ages, but in modified forms. The older cases are comparatively less concentrated among homosexual and bisexual males or among IV drug abusers; they are comparatively less concentrated in minority populations or among men rather than women. Similar modifications may take place in the total society if the epidemic continues to spread through heterosexual contact beyond its original enclaves. In such respects, a deeper understanding of the current experiences of older people with AIDS might provide a useful scenario for informing both preventive efforts and estimates of societal trends for the future.

Aging and the Natural History of the Disease

Past and possible future trends in the age patterns of HIV infection and AIDS can be understood only by examining the underlying dynamic processes. AIDS is not an isolated event that occurs at a single moment of time in a body that is changeless. AIDS is, rather, a protracted disease, which coincides with a major segment of the individual's life course. While the HIV virus is developing, the infected individuals—until they die—are growing older. Thus those now infected who are in their forties may have passed age 50 before being diagnosed with AIDS, and those now infected who are in their sixties may have passed age 70. These two sets of dynamic processes, AIDS and aging, running concurrently over a person's lifetime, are continually interacting with one another. In addition, they share an important common feature: Both sets of processes are marked by heterogeneity, as individuals differ widely both in expression of the disease and in the ways they grow old.

HIV Infection and Biopsychosocial Aging Processes

A great deal is known about the processes of aging, and much is being learned about the mechanisms linking these processes with many forms of illness and disability (see, e.g., Riley, 1983a). Aging is a complex set of processes, which include social, psychological, and biological changes: For example, associated with aging are tendencies for vulnerability to disease to increase, stressful life events to multiply, or behavioral responses to become slower.

Knowledge is also accumulating about the progression of HIV infection from first exposure up until death (Redfield & Burke, 1988; see also American Public Health Association, 1988). Once infected, it is reported that the majority show some evidence of progressive immunodeficiency and, in the absence of effective therapy, most seem likely to develop AIDS. However, the period between infection and onset of symptoms can be very long, as the body's immune system defends against the virus. During this interval, which can last in some individuals for as much as 7 to 10 years, the infected person can look healthy and remain asymptomatic, before the immune system finally breaks down and the symptoms of AIDS become apparent. Moreover, as AZT and other forms of treatment are utilized, the entire process may be prolonged. Yet, during this asymptomatic interval, the infected person, often unwittingly, can still transmit the infection to others.

What is not known is how these two sets of processes, aging and HIV infection, interact with each other, although there are a few straws in the wind. For example, low levels of awareness of AIDS among older people may make them even more vulnerable than younger people, as in couples where one partner erroneously believes the relationship to be entirely monogamous, or where one has unknowingly been infected through blood transfusion. In another example, an analysis of transfusion cases[10] where the date of exposure to HIV was known showed a tendency for the time period between exposure and diagnosis of AIDS to decrease with increasing age of the patient exposed. This finding raises the provocative question of whether declines in immune function, which are known to be associated with aging, may in some way be connected with age-related increases in susceptibility to AIDS. In still another example from a large study of homosexually active men (Ostrow, Monjan, Joseph, et al., in press), a man's self-reported physical symptoms rather than HIV antibody status predicted psychological distress. By contrast, other researchers have shown that older people are comparatively more likely to attribute symptoms to their age rather than to disease, and thus might well never report to a physician such AIDS-related symptoms as excessive fatigue.

Heterogeneity of the Processes

Another parallel between aging and HIV lies in the heterogeneity of both processes. It is well established that individuals vary widely in the ways in which they grow old: they range from those who lead long, healthy, effective, and fulfilling lives to those who succumb early in life to ill health, poor levels of functioning, loneliness, and withdrawal from affairs. Similarly, there is wide variation among individuals in the nature, timing, and manifestations of the HIV virus. Over time, an infected person may begin to develop such symptoms as weight loss, excessive fatigue, headaches, or swollen lymph glands; and, once diagnosed with AIDS, the symptoms may include special

[10] Data especially prepared by the Centers for Disease Control (CDC), but based on very small samples, and without correction for shortened life-expectancy at the oldest ages.

forms of pneumonia or cancer, neurological signs and symptoms as the brain becomes implicated, as well as many more familiar diseases such as tuberculosis (Redfield & Burke, 1988).

Such parallels point to the potential for using existing knowledge about aging and other diseases to increase understanding of the social and psychological factors that may affect HIV infection in older individuals, and may influence the means of preventing or coping with the disease.

In sum, in the older population AIDS is now just beginning. Only one-tenth of AIDS cases today occur in people aged 50 and over, in contrast to one quarter of the United States population being in that age category. In several respects the current situation of older people with AIDS provides a wide frontier for prevention of further infection. The many older homosexual and bisexual men and transfusion recipients who are already infected can, without adequate precautions, carry the virus to their life partners and other female or male sexual partners. Yet older people are comparatively unaware, uninformed, and unconcerned about AIDS. The key attitude is, "It can't happen to me." The challenge for prevention is serious indeed.

ORGANIZATION OF THE BOOK

Many aspects of these relationships among AIDS, the aging society, and individual aging processes are examined in the following chapters in this book. Each chapter covers a range of topics, with the same point often examined repeatedly, but in different contexts. Despite their diversity, the chapters are organized in three main parts according to their major contributions to the book, with the parts focused respectively on risk factors and prevention, care, and societal consequences. In addition, each chapter raises questions about the future course of the epidemic and makes suggestions for an agenda of needed research, and the appended references afford a wide-ranging bibliography for readers interested in further exploration of particular topics.

In this section of the introductory chapter, a preview of each of the later chapters will serve to locate its central objectives within the book as a whole, as well as to indicate occasional points which, in the judgment of the editors, need further development. Further introductory commentary by Maddox and Maddox appears in Chapter 2, "The Complementarity of Psychosocial and Biomedical Research on AIDS." These authors stress the importance—too widely neglected—of the behavioral and social factors that interact with the biomedical factors in influencing the etiology, course, and outcomes of AIDS, and they emphasize age and the life course as critical mediators of these influences.

Risk Factors and Prevention

The four chapters in Part II of the book examine many aspects of the existing knowledge about the risk factors for transmission of the HIV virus, and about measures taken, or neglected, for preventing the spread of the epidemic. In Chapter 3, Levy and Albrecht, of the School of Public Health at the University of Illinois at Chicago present a broad background "Review of Research on Sexual and AIDS-Related Attitudes and Behaviors." In describing the relevant literature, they point both to the neglect and to the far-reaching implications of middle-aged and older people in studies of human sexuality. They report the many ways in which older people's AIDS-related knowledge, attitudes, and behaviors differ from those of younger people. In addition to focusing on what is known about sex and AIDS among older homosexual and bisexual males, they provide information about older people's role in transmission through IV drug abuse, blood transfusion, and heterosexual contacts.

Also providing essential background for the book as a whole is Chapter 4, "The Social Epidemiology of AIDS and HIV Infection among Older Americans," by Stall, Catania, and Pollack. These authors present a series of tables that show differences by age in the distribution and sources of transmission of the new AIDS cases reported to the Centers for Disease Control (CDC) over the years from pre-1982 through 1987. These tables are so invaluable that they are cross-referenced in nearly every chapter of the book—the only misfortune being that, because of the change in the CDC definition of AIDS, direct comparisons cannot be made with the cumulative data including 1988 as shown in Tables 1.1 and 1.2 above. In their chapter, Stall and associates outline a possible model for estimating the needs for care of older persons with AIDS, which indicates that older people will almost certainly constitute a substantial minority of the probable future caseload. Moreover, they report findings from a study of gay and bisexual men in San Francisco showing the extent, sources, and changes in behavioral risk. Treating AIDS as an "age-defined disease," they identify age-related targets for prevention efforts and set out a research agenda for examining the place of older AIDS victims in the care setting.

The critical distinction between AIDS as the diagnosable disease and HIV as the often hidden virus is clearly drawn in Chapter 5, "HIV Transmission Risks of Older Heterosexuals and Gays." The authorship, by Catania and six collaborators who include the authors of Chapter 4 as well as others with varied affiliations at the University of California at San Francisco, symbolizes the high degree of communication among students of social and behavioral aspects of AIDS. These investigators, who deal with primary prevention of HIV infection, describe two comparatively neglected sources of transmission of the virus: blood transfusions and heterosexual relations, both of which are important at the later ages. Reasoning from the diagnosed AIDS cases (for which the only data are reported), they emphasize that the long lag time between infection and the onset of symptoms means that the data on AIDS cases reflect infection patterns of as much as 5 to 7 years earlier. Transfusion-related AIDS cases, the second largest risk group (after homosexual and bisexual males) among people aged 50 and over, have been increasing sharply in relative importance since 1982. Although blood screening for HIV was initiated in 1985, the potential spread through sexual transmission from those already infected is incalculable. AIDS cases attributable to heterosexual transmission, which we see as the ultimate key to the future scope of the epidemic, are still relatively few, but they have shown a steadily increasing trend among older people. As a further contribution of this chapter, the authors make use of existing psychosocial knowledge and theories about behavior change to formulate a model of reduction in AIDS risk.

In Chapter 6, Levy and Albrecht describe another translation of social science principles for use in understanding of AIDS, in this instance to "Methodological Considerations in Research on Sexual Behavior and AIDS among Older People." This chapter discusses methodological problems and possible research strategies inherent in investigations focused on highly sensitive subject matter, on older people, and on people not only as individuals but also as partners in intimate personal relationships. The authors touch on such topics as special populations to be studied, units of analysis, sampling, data collection procedures and instruments, handling of refusals and missing values, and ethical dilemmas relating to confidentiality and informed consent.

Care

The chapters in Part III shift the major focus from prevention of AIDS to care of the afflicted. These chapters consider older people as caregivers to relatives with AIDS, or as AIDS patients needing care, or as themselves users of long-term care whose traditional resources are threatened by competing demands from this new epidemic. Each of the two chapters in this part demonstrate once again the relevance of the social sciences to the understanding of AIDS: Chapter 7 applies existing sociological concepts and models of the "illness career," and Chapter 8 applies to AIDS patients knowledge that is available in the literature on long-term care of older people.

Chapter 7, "On the Relevance of Social Science Concepts and Perspectives," is written by a varied set of collaborators, McKinlay, Skinner, J. Riley, and Zablotsky. It illustrates how such scientifically defined concepts as "stigma," "sick role," or "labeling" can bring to bear a wealth of disparate knowledge and thought not only in interpreting the implications of findings about AIDS, but also in using the accumulated knowledge as bases for designing appropriate interventions. The authors point to the historical parallels between AIDS and other epidemics, recalling that biological science is not a necessary prerequisite for effective social action and public health programs. They also show how sociological perspectives help to illuminate the attitudes, behaviors, and social relationships of older AIDS patients and the treatment of these patients as embedded within the formal and informal systems of health care.

In Chapter 8, Crystal makes use of the parallel between "Persons with AIDS and Older People: Common Long-Term Concerns." He examines issues of organization, delivery, and outcome of long-term care as they affect both patient populations: those with AIDS, and that minority of older people who are afflicted with chronic illness or disability. Much that has already been learned about health services research and programs for the frail elderly can be usefully applied to care of people with AIDS. Moreover, there is an interplay involved: as AIDS patients utilize models of long-term care originally established for older people, the new and innovative models developed in response to the AIDS epidemic can, in turn, inform improved health care options available to older people.

Societal Consequences

Unlike the immediate need for prevention of AIDS and the pressing demands for appropriate care and support at each stage of the natural history of the disease, the impact of the epidemic on society raises long-range questions for the future. Part IV of the book begins to raise just a few of these larger questions.

Chapter 9, by Manton and Singer, deals with "Forecasting the Impact of the AIDS Epidemic on Elderly Populations." In a highly technical exposition, yet understandable by the layman, these two leading experts in mathematical modeling explain why the methods of simple extrapolation currently used by most students of AIDS are inappropriate. They call for development of new types of models, more suitable to the special circumstances of the AIDS epidemic. Such models are biosocially realistic, can represent the uncertainty of the phenomena to be described, and can integrate data from multiple sources. A three-pronged research agenda is set forth for forecasting: (1) both quantitative and qualitative aspects of the future course of the AIDS epidemic among older adults; (2) the impact of increased AIDS-related demand for acute and long-term health care services; and (3) the collection and compilation of data necessary for making such forecasts.

Looking toward current and future changes in the society as a whole, Chapter 10 deals with "The Social Consequences of the AIDS Epidemic: A Challenge for the Social Sciences." Written by Ergas, who works with other scholars enlisted by the Social Science Research Council in New York City, the chapter gives a farreaching overview of predictable modes of social and cultural adaptations and of ensuing policy issues. It begins with an historical view of the ways in which epidemics have shaped and been shaped by structures of social, economic, and political life (medical science is included in these structures). Ergas touches on the accentuation of social cleavages, as the AIDS epidemic has exacerbated the disadvantages of minorities and has highlighted sexuality as a "liberal–conservative" issue. Additional topics that are covered include the economic burden, the mobilization of support groups, and the implications for education and for health care facilities. The aim of the chapter is to develop a research agenda that can inform the coping strategies in society so as to forestall negative outcomes, while identifying the positive innovations to which health crises sometimes give rise.

In the concluding "Notes for the Future: Research, Care, Prevention, Public Policy," Ory and Zablotsky highlight selected research themes from the areas covered in the set of chapters in the book as a whole. Returning to the central objective of the book, this final chapter contributes to an integrated understanding of what we know, what we need to know, and some implications for future public policy and professional practice.

APPLICABILITY OF SOCIAL AND BEHAVIORAL SCIENCE

Clearly, then, much of what we know and need to know about AIDS among older people is identified in one or another form in the chapters of this book. One theme running through these chapters is of such vital importance to an understanding of HIV and AIDS as to be underscored in this introductory chapter: namely, the relevance not only of the biomedical, but also of the social and behavioral, sciences.

As several of the authors indicate, future research can be enhanced, current understandings deepened, and interventions guided by synthesizing and applying principles and knowledge already available in the social and behavioral sciences. Thus care of AIDS patients can be informed by existing studies of long-term care of older people; contextual influences on the natural history of AIDS can be clarified through knowledge of the illness career; studies of sensitive topics such as sexual behavior or sexually transmitted diseases can be benefited through established procedures of sociological research; forecasts can be improved through use of models adequately grounded in the social sciences; and the societal consequences of the epidemic can be illuminated by the principles of social and cultural dynamics.

In addition to the examples cited throughout the book, there are numerous other scientific strands that can make noteworthy contributions to understanding AIDS in an aging society. Among them, though not discussed in detail here, are aspects of the extensive knowledge and theory in medical sociology;[11] and the pertinent sociological findings on diffusion of innovation, on mass communication and persuasion, and on behavior change. Three relevant social science strands cannot be overlooked, however: the relation to AIDS of the sociology of age, the cross-cultural perspective, and research on social networks and social relationships.

Age, Aging, and AIDS

The sociology of age (cf. Riley, 1987; Riley, Foner, & Waring, 1988), which distinguishes between a cross-sectional approach and a cohort approach, informs understanding of the AIDS epidemic. Each approach is appropriate for examining particular aspects of the disease, although inappropriate use leads to fallacious interpretations.

In this book, primary attention is paid to the cross-sectional approach for describing age differences. For example, in Tables 1.1 and 1.2 above, numbers and kinds of people who differ in age—that is, who belong in different age categories or age strata—are compared. Cross-sectional views have specific uses for certain objectives of this book. They can be used, for example, to examine whether or not there is "intergenerational equity" in allocation of health care resources to older people with Alzheimer's disease rather than to younger people with AIDS. Sequential cross-sections are needed for examining societal trends, such as trends in concentrations of the disease in particular segments of the population. For example, among very old people, the majority of whom are women, will the prevalence of AIDS remain higher among men?

Of particular relevance for the concern of this book with AIDS in an aging society are cross-sectional analyses of the critical societal changes in the age composition of the population. The population of the United States already confronts staggering problems because the proportion of older people is continually increasing at dramatic rates; if the AIDS epidemic were to produce sufficient deaths among younger people, it could compound these problems. The predictable consequences of any accelerated aging of the population would reverberate through the social structure, affecting families, the work force, migration patterns, and the many other social and cultural institutions described by Ergas in Chapter 10. These consequences could only exacerbate the current disjunctures between the rising proportions of older people and declining opportunities for them to perform useful and rewarding social roles.[12]

[11] Much theory and knowledge of relevance to HIV and AIDS derives from the field of medical sociology. See, e.g., Ory and Bond, 1989; also McKinlay, McKinlay, and Beaglehole, forthcoming.
[12] This disjuncture, which I have described as "structural lag" (e.g. Riley, Foner, & Waring, 1988), has implications not only for the consequences of an AIDS epidemic, but also for issues of both prevention and care of the disease.

Equally as important as the cross-section approach, but for quite different purposes in understanding how age is implicated in AIDS, is the cohort approach. When a cohort is defined as a set of individuals born at the same time, this approach examines the different ways in which members of different cohorts grow up and grow older. Within each cohort, when the lives of individuals are traced longitudinally, the heterogeneity among these lives is observed to increase with advancing age (Dannefer, 1987); thus the many factors affecting both prevention and care of AIDS are even more complex among older than among younger people. Failure to take this heterogeneity into account produces the widespread "fallacy of averages." As different cohorts succeed one another through different periods of historical time, members of these different cohorts grow old in different ways, because society is continually changing around them. Failure to take these cohort differences into account leads to the widespread "life-course fallacy," that is, erroneously assuming that cross-sectional age differences can be interpreted as describing the process of aging.

The power of the cohort approach has crept into popular thought through experience with the "baby boom cohort," which, as everyone knows, will ultimately increase the proportions of older people in the society. However, the most striking increase will not occur until 2020, a date beyond the probable lifetime of anyone now infected with HIV. As a more relevant example of the cohort approach, many members of the cohort of persons who in 1988 are still in their forties (born in the 1940s), if recently infected, will have reached age 50 and over before the virus surfaces as the AIDS disease. Yet, as compared with the earlier cohort born in the 1930s or before whom we now study as "AIDS cases aged 50 and over," that more recent cohort will have had different experiences and will predictably be different in many ways. For example, it is already known that members of this more recent cohort have learned earlier in life to be aware of their personal risks of exposure to the AIDS virus, are more likely to have discussed AIDS with a friend or relative, and are more knowledgeable about how HIV infection can be prevented or how the disease becomes manifest (Dawson, 1988).

To broaden the temporal scope of such examples, the cohorts who were leading their lives during the Black Death of the 14th century, or during the influenza epidemics of 1918 and subsequent years, experienced both similarities with, and differences from, the cohorts growing older during the AIDS epidemic today—experiences from which significant lessons might be gleaned. As Joshua Lederberg puts it (1988a), "our stratagems on malaria, gonococcus, and human immunodeficiency virus are all confounded by the poorly understood capacity of the viruses to undergo further antigenic evolution." As successive cohorts of human beings grow older, it is not only society that is changing, but also the microbes "that remain our competitors of last resort for dominion of the planet" (p. 684). Much is to be learned from the sociology of science, not only about the current HIV epidemic, but also about how to prepare for probable future epidemics (Lederberg, 1988b). Historical experience describes, for example, the response to sudden epidemics through adaptation of health care institutions, incorporation of scientific developments into medical practice, or practices of producing and distributing vaccines and treatments once they are discovered.

Cross-Cultural Perspectives on AIDS

Older people are parts of social systems, some small and intimate, others worldwide, and, just as fuller understanding of AIDS requires extending the sociotemporal scope of the analysis, it also requires extending the spatial scope. A great deal is to be learned from cross-cultural analyses of older people's experiences with this disease, especially because situations vary from those in which the epidemic is fully established to those only now beginning to report occasional cases.

Though special social and behavioral studies of older populations remain to be done, considerable research has been reported on HIV and AIDS in other countries throughout the world. Reports from the World Health Organization (WHO) in Geneva (Mann et al., 1988), where surveillance of AIDS is coordinated for all regions of the world, indicate that HIV was spreading silently and extensively in the 1970s and perhaps even earlier, although the actual origin of HIV is still not known with any certainty.

Three patterns of AIDS are identified in the WHO reports. Pattern I characterizes those industrialized countries having large numbers of AIDS cases and resembles closely the epidemiology described in this book for the United States. Pattern II, which is currently found in parts of Africa and in some Latin American countries, particularly in the Caribbean, contrasts with Pattern I in that it predominates among heterosexuals, and the numbers of infected females and males are approximately equal. Pattern III prevails in areas of Eastern Europe, North Africa, and the Middle East, where HIV was probably introduced early in the 1980s and few cases have so far been reported.

The continent hardest hit by the pandemic is Africa. Here all three infection patterns are to be found (see Miller & Rockwell, 1988), and the consequences can be fully examined. It is in the countries of central and east Africa in particular that, with deaths concentrated among those in their twenties and thirties, a "hollowing out" occurs in the age composition of the population. This hollowing out can affect the leadership core, as well as those components of the labor force engaged in agriculture, the military, or other forms of work requiring youthful strength and vigor. As Kenneth Prewitt (1988, p. ix) puts it:

> In complex ways AIDS disrupts the economic and social development of Africa—the loss of trained personnel, the deflection of scarce resources, the strain on public health and education systems, the reduction of tourist revenue, and the potential political unrest resulting from a pressing social problem.

What, then, are the implications of a full-fledged epidemic for those in their middle and later years? On the one hand, if older people remain free of AIDS, will they be needed to replace the young in productive activities? Or, on the other hand, will the societal surroundings be so disrupted as to be unable to meet even the minimum needs of those few elderly who do have AIDS? Clearly, there is much to be learned from other societies, where the wide variations in the forms and the inclusiveness of the epidemic provide a laboratory for investigating the processes through which AIDS implicates the lives of people at every age, including those in their middle and later years.

AIDS and Social Relationships

Turning from the macrolevel society to the smaller social systems in which older people are embedded, it is a central tenet of sociology that everyone belongs in interpersonal networks. Individuals cannot be understood apart from their social relationships and interactions, or from the processes affecting them through the small groups, such as families or neighborhoods, of which they are members. In the words of John Donne, "No man is an island, entire of itself."

The applicability to AIDS is obvious. Sexual contact typically involves more than one person, and the patterns of sexual conduct and disease transmission are likely to be influenced by both partners to the sexual transaction and the bond between them (National Opinion Research Center, 1987). Ironically, however, much of the research on AIDS is atomistic, focusing on discrete individuals, or on aggregates of individuals. The concept of social relationships, so central to sociological theory, has proved difficult to implement in large-scale, systematic surveys (in contrast to its success in guiding in-depth studies of single networks or single communities).

Nevertheless, various methods of relational analysis are available for use in sociological studies of AIDS based on large population samples (e.g., Coleman, 1986; Marsden & Laumann, 1984; Riley, 1983b; and for an analysis of earlier work, see Riley, 1963). Of immediate relevance is a design for a cross-sectional survey of sexual behavior and AIDS, developed by the staff of the National Opinion Research Center (NORC) at the University of Chicago. This design incorporates both a conceptual framework and a research procedure for analysis of networks. As outlined in the original research proposal (National Opinion

Research Center, 1987), the research unit is envisioned as a possible "core quartet" consisting of the focal actor (the respondent in the survey), a primary partner role, and two secondary partner roles, one female and one male. Translated into survey operations, each respondent is to be asked to describe persons in each of these four roles—wherever there are such persons in the respondent's network. So ideal a design for research rarely finds opportunity to be fully implemented; but, as aspects of the plan are tested, the experience will become a model for further research on this and other epidemics.

There are many other examples, of course, of the translation into research of social science concepts that are relevant to AIDS. Among them is the life-course perspective, for which numerous procedures of longitudinal analysis are available. The NORC design also aims to combine network analysis with a life-course approach, conceiving of each single sexual event as embedded in the context of other antecedent, concurrent, and impending events.

In sum, increasingly sophisticated study of AIDS in an aging society need not begin *de novo.* In applying what we know, and in learning what we need to know, pertinent social science knowledge, conceptual frameworks, and research methods are already at hand.

CONCLUSION

In line with the central objective of this book, the chapters provide numerous and diverse clues to information already available about AIDS in an aging society. They describe the relationship between AIDS and aging. They deal with many details of risk factors and problems and possibilities for prevention. They show the parallelism between systems of long-term care, both formal and informal, for older people and for people dying from AIDS. They describe methods of forecasting the future course of the epidemic and outline the possible impact of an epidemic on social institutions and structures.

At the same time, the chapters emphasize what we still need to know. Among the great unknowns are the ratios between reported cases of AIDS and the still hidden cases of HIV infection: very rough estimates as of 1988 indicate a ratio in the United States of some 70,000 to a million or a million and half (Heyward & Curran, 1988), and in the world of 250,000 to 5 or 10 million (Mann et al., 1988). It is these HIV cases that set the stage for the future, a stage on which effective measures of prevention and of long-term care can strongly influence the outcomes. It is here that social science knowledge, principles, and methods have direct relevance. In particular, the sociology of age and medical sociology have equipped us to address challenges posed by HIV infection and AIDS in an aging society. And, in turn, solutions to the AIDS crisis may feed back into the social science literature and produce unseen benefits in relation to other illnesses and other epidemics.

Running throughout the book is the central theme to which this chapter is addressed: that in scientific research and public concern with AIDS, the middle-aged and older people constitute the overlooked segment of the population. Little effort has been made to educate them about AIDS or to provide facilities to help them in prevention or in care.[13] Even older people themselves are unaware of the dangers. Few seem ready to make use of whatever techniques are generally available for self-protection, or of counseling, tests, or, if needed, early diagnosis and treatment. Few have so far had the direct experience of caring for a relative who is dying from AIDS.

However, within this older population, the epidemic is not yet fully entrenched. There is still time for preventive efforts—as much time for this segment as there was back in the early stages of the epidemic for the population as a whole. And there is still time to reexamine the formal and the informal systems of long-term care, which must now accommodate not only frail older people, but also people of all ages who are afflicted with AIDS.

The final chapter of the volume, "Notes for the Future: Research, Care, Prevention, Public Policy," looks ahead toward meeting some of these challenges. It outlines types of research that can provide the knowledge base for needed interventions. And it points to the kinds of interventions that can help to overcome the neglect of older people, can guide prevention, and can enhance the care of both the frail elderly and people of all ages who have been or may be stricken by AIDS.

REFERENCES

American Public Health Association. 1988. "Casual Contact and the Risk of HIV Infection." Report of Special Initiative on AIDS. 1015 Fifteenth St. NW, Washington, D.C. 20005.

Centers for Disease Control. 1987. "Human Immunodeficiency Virus Infection in the United States: A Review of Current Knowledge." *Morbidity and Mortality Weekly Report* 36 (sup. no. S-6).

Coleman, James S. 1986. "Micro-Foundations and Macro-Social Theory." Pp. 345–63 in *Approaches to Social Theory,* edited by S. Lindberg, J. Coleman, and S. Nowak. New York: Russell Sage Foundation.

Dannefer, Dale. 1987. "Aging as Intracohort Differentiation: Accentuation, the Matthew Effect, and the Life Course." *Sociological Forum* 2 (spring):211–36.

Dawson, Deborah A. 1988. "AIDS Knowledge and Attitudes for May and June, 1988." *NCHS advance data* 160 (September 26). DHHS Publication No. (PHS)88-1250.

[13] While there are many organizations providing service to older people in general, or advocating their causes, these seem to be paying little specific heed to people with AIDS.

Heyward, William L., and James W. Curran. 1988. "The Epidemiology of AIDS in the U.S." *Scientific American* 259 (4):72–81.

Lederberg, Joshua. 1988a. "Medical Science, Infectious Disease, and the Unity of Mankind." *Journal of the American Medical Association* 260(5):684–5.

———. 1988b. "Pandemic as a Natural Evolutionary Phenomenon." *Social Research* 55(3), Autumn:344–359.

Mann, Jonathan M., James Chin, Peter Piot, and Thomas Quinn. 1988. "The International Epidemiology of AIDS." *Scientific American* 259(4):82–9.

Marsden, P., and Edward O. Laumann. 1984. "Mathematical Ideas in Social Structural Analysis." *Journal of Mathematical Sociology* 10:271–94.

McKinlay, John B., Sonja M. McKinlay, and Robert Beaglehole. (forthcoming). "Trends in Death and Disease and the Contribution of Medical Measures." In *Handbook of Medical Sociology* (4th ed.), edited by H.E. Freeman and S. Levine. New Jersey: Prentice-Hall.

Miller, Norman, and Richard C. Rockwell. 1988. *AIDS In Africa: The Social and Policy Impact.* Lewiston, NY: The Edwin Mellen Press.

National Opinion Research Center (NORC), University of Chicago. 1987. *Technical Proposal, Social and Behavioral Aspects of Health and Fertility-Related Behavior* (unpublished).

Ory, Marcia, and Kathleen Bond. 1989. "Introduction: Health Care for an Aging Society." Pp. 1–24 in *Aging and Health Care: Social Science and Policy Perspectives,* edited by M. Ory and K. Bond. London: Tavistock.

Ostrow, David G., Andrew Monjan, Jill Joseph, et al. (in press). "HIV-Related Symptoms and Psychological Functioning in a Cohort of Homosexual Men." *American Journal of Pyschiatry.*

Pifer, Alan, and Lydia Bronte. 1986. *Our Aging Society: Paradox and Promise.* New York: W.W. Norton.

Prewitt, Kenneth. 1988. Foreword: "AIDS In Africa: The Triple Disaster." Pp. ix–xii in *AIDS In Africa: The Social and Policy Impact*, edited by N. Miller and R.C. Rockwell. Lewiston, NY: The Edwin Mellen Press.

Public Health Reports. 1988. "Report of the Second Public Health Service AIDS Prevention and Control Conference." *Journal of the U.S. Public Health Service.* Volume 103, Sup. 1.

Redfield, Robert R., and Donald S. Burke. 1988. "HIV Infection: The Clinical Picture." *Scientific American* 259(4):90–8.

Riley, Matilda White. 1963. *Sociological Research (Vol. I, Unit 12).* New York: Harcourt, Brace, Jovanovich.

———. 1983a. "Cancer and the Life Course." Pp. 25–32 in *Prevention and Treatment of Cancer in the Elderly* edited by R. Yancik et al. New York: Raven Press.

———. 1983b. "The Family in an Aging Society: A Matrix of Latent Relationships." *Journal of Family Issues* 4(3):439–454.

———. 1987. "Aging, Health, and Social Change: An Overview." Pp. 1–14 in *Perspectives on Behavioral Medicine*, vol. IV, *The Aging Dimension,* edited by M.W. Riley, J.D. Matarazzo, and A. Baum. Hillsdale, NJ: Lawrence Erlbaum Associates, Inc.

Riley, Matilda White, Anne Foner, and Joan Waring. 1988. "Sociology of Age." Pp. 243–90 in *Handbook of Sociology,* edited by N. Smelser. New York: Sage.

Turner, Charles F., Heather G. Miller, and Lincon E. Moses (editors). 1989. *AIDS, Sexual Behavior and Intravenous Drug Use.* Washington, D.C.: National Academy Press.

CHAPTER 2

The Complementarity of Psychosocial and Biomedical Research on AIDS

George L. Maddox and G. David Maddox

Our point of departure for scanning relevant literature and for conceptualizing problems posed by AIDS was to ask whether and how age and the life course are discussed as relevant issues. We also asked whether and how behavioral and social factors were perceived to interact with biomedical factors in explaining the etiology, course, and outcomes of AIDS. We found that neither set of questions has yet been answered adequately and concluded that much work needs to be done in which aging and life-course issues and in which behavioral and social aspects of illness are addressed.

The rapidly growing scientific literature on AIDS in the last several years is distinctive in several ways. First, its predominant focus is biomedical, a characterization confirmed by the collected reprints from two prestigious journals, *The New England Journal of Medicine* (1987) and *Science* (Kulstad, 1986). Second, interest in psychosocial and life-course variables has been modest in spite of a strong contrary recommendation of the Institute of Medicine (1986, 1988) stressing the importance of nonbiomedical factors. Third, the sociocultural embeddedness of health and illness is illustrated particularly well by the controversies regarding morality, civil liberties, and science policy provoked by AIDS in both lay and scientific media (e.g., Brandt, 1985, 1988; Osborn, 1988; Panem, 1988; Shilts, 1987; Willis, 1986).

We find three compelling reasons for introducing life-course and psychosocial perspectives into research on AIDS. We go beyond a declaration of strong interest in these perspectives to argue for the opportunity of the social and behavioral sciences to make contributions (1) to the prevention and epidemiology of AIDS as age-related phenomena; (2) to a better understanding of the ways in which persons with AIDS or at high risk to contract the disease can be helped through psychosocial as well as biomedical intervention; and (3) to appreciation of the far-reaching societal reactions to a multifaceted disease process that does not reduce easily to biomedical explanation but that benefits from a long-term psychosocial perspective. Thus our reading of this literature on AIDS anticipates several of the points developed further in this volume.

REAFFIRMING A MULTIDISCIPLINARY PERSPECTIVE

The scientific study of human aging has, from its modern origins over four decades ago, been distinctively characterized by its multidisciplinary perspective. Few significant problems in human aging reduce simply to the theoretical models or research methods of any single discipline. In 1974 the United States Congress acknowledged this characterization in the distinctive mandate given at the National Institutes of Health to the National Institute on Aging (NIA). NIA's mandate specifically recognized the complementary contributions of the behavioral and social sciences and the biomedical sciences.

AIDS, particularly in relation to age, is a striking example of a type of problem threatening health and survival that can best be understood by conceptualizing the issues to focus on the complementarity of psychosocial and biomedical factors. However, the temptation to view AIDS as primarily or exclusively a biomedical problem has obviously been great. Such a view of disease instructs investigators to identify a causal agent, develop a test to identify the presence of the causal agent, and produce a vaccine or other biological agent to immunize individuals at risk or reduce the effects of the disease. In the social history of medicine in the United States, the biomedical approach has prevailed, and public confidence and substantial financial support for biomedical research has followed. Yet numerous commentaries illustrate how the preferred biomedical model, which has been characterized as a search for "the silver bullet," has not always worked (Brandt, 1985, 1988; McKinlay, McKinlay, & Beaglehole, 1988; Willis, 1986). A relevant and instructive illustration of the limits of a narrow biomedical conceptualization of disease process and responses to disease is found in sexually transmitted disease. The history of syphilis over the past century illustrates how medical science can identify viral agents that it may be able to contain but not prevent; it also illustrates how the transmission of viral agents is deeply embedded in behavior patterns resistant to both rationalistic and moralistic preachments about risk (Brandt, 1985; Metropolitan Life, 1986).

BEHAVIORAL EPIDEMIOLOGY AND PREVENTION OF AIDS

If prevention is the strategy of choice for coping with the AIDS epidemic, the epidemiology of AIDS demands greater attention. Evidence accumulated by the Centers for Disease Control (CDC) and others since 1980 has documented the spread of AIDS and characterized the disease with increasing precision (Booth, 1988; Curran et al., 1988). We know a great deal about many basic risk factors, particularly about the risk associated with certain male homosexual practices, IV drug use, and pre-1985 blood transfusions. Evidence is accumulating (at least in today's limited statistics) that AIDS apparently is not spread easily through ordinary social interaction or casual contact. And we know that while the risk of AIDS is highest in the middle adult years, CDC reports that a persistent 10% of new AIDS cases each year are 50 years of age and older.

Population Estimates

What we do not know about the epidemiology of AIDS is as impressive and, perhaps, more consequential socially than what we know. For example, epidemiological evidence has continued to be fundamentally flawed by an inability to secure reliable and generalizable information about how exposure to the AIDS virus translates into seropositivity and seropositivity progresses into AIDS or related opportunistic infection. The evidence has remained flawed in part from technical limitations in the reliable identification of seropositivity. The highly emotional public response to AIDS, which has been a mixture of prudent concern, personal fear, and often moral revulsion, has largely prevented adequate sampling of general and special populations, save in special situations where, for example, routine testing of newborns for HIV is possible. Indirect approaches to sampling problems (e.g., using military inductees, blood donors, patients in clinics for sexually transmitted diseases) have proved to be less than adequate (Felman & Johnson, 1986; Janes, 1986; Quinn et al., 1988). Consequently, estimates of current and projected AIDS cases necessarily and realistically have very broad confidence limits (Lambert, 1987). The chapters in this volume document just how uncertain the scientific community remains about the current and future incidence and prevalence of seropositivity and AIDS in the general population, although there is general agreement that the risk of AIDS is unacceptably high. The chapter by Stall, Catania, and colleagues, which argues that AIDS is an age-defined epidemic, is particularly pertinent.

Latency and Aging

The latency of AIDS following exposure is, in our view, a particularly important issue for understanding the complementarity of biomedical and psychosocial approaches and the salience of age and life course as epidemiological variables. Existing research is especially unconvincing regarding the timing of the process that translates exposure into seropositivity into AIDS. Yet the timing of this process coincides with the aging of the person involved. Basic sampling problems prevent any definitive description of the disease process at this time. For example, the date of infection can rarely be reliably specified except for the person with AIDS who was exposed to the virus by blood transfusion, where some evidence suggests a mean latency time (from exposure to diagnosis of AIDS) of less than 10 years (Curran et al., 1988; Medley et al., 1987). Whether this estimate can be extrapolated to latency for persons exposed in other ways is unclear.

Limited evidence does suggest population heterogeneity in the risk of exposure, the latency following exposure, and the risk of translating exposure into AIDS. Interestingly, estimates of average latency following exposure have tended to increase as the epidemic has progressed. But one still has a choice regarding whether the best estimate of average latency is 4 years or 8 years or 15 years. Perhaps the answer is "all of the above," depending on the particular subpopulation under consideration. Latency is almost certainly longer than many current estimates and will vary among subpopulations. As a case in point, insofar as AIDS is basically a problem of immunodeficiency, and the efficiency of the immune system is known to be partially a function of age, one is not surprised to encounter in the literature on AIDS occasional conjectures that AIDS latency should be shortest among the very young and the very old.

Thus the meaning of age as a variable in epidemiologic research on AIDS has been incidental, not central. CDC regularly reports the distribution of AIDS by age, including (as noted above) the fact that a relatively stable 10% of diagnosed cases are 50 years of age and older. Interest in the systematic analysis of age as a variable is deflected in part by the awareness that as of 1987 some 68% of the newly reported AIDS cases are between the ages of 13 and 39, and another 22% are between the ages of 40 and 49. While the public probably associates AIDS with youthfulness or young adulthood, the observed distribution includes a substantial number of cases in middle and late adulthood. As a practical matter, then, if one notes the number of AIDS cases in late middle life, and factors in an uncertain but undoubtedly long latency of the AIDS virus, a significant number of future AIDS cases will inevitably be among late-middle-aged and older adults.

MOBILIZING SOCIAL SUPPORT AND CARE OVER THE LIFE COURSE

Persuasive research on coping with the challenges to health and well-being in later life has established the critical importance of social support (Cohen & Syme, 1985; House et al., 1988). The importance of social support is found in research that suggests supportive relationships may have an "immunizing" function in detoxifying a variety of stressors. This research also documents the modifying effect that social support has on adaptive behavior when one is challenged by stressful events. We would generalize these observations to show that informal social supports, which constitute the bulk of care for dependent older persons, are critically important in responding to most stressors and over the entire life course.

We looked with interest, therefore, for any systematic study of social support mobilization for persons exposed to AIDS or identified as AIDS patients. Our interest was driven by the prospect that, in an environment highly prejudicial against homosexuality and IV drug use, persons with AIDS might be at high risk for being denied normally expected levels of social support, particularly support from the most common source of such support, which is from persons related by kinship. (See also the discussions of these issues in the chapters in this volume by Crystal and by McKinlay et al.)

Our search for evidence regarding AIDS and social support identified very little systematic evidence. There were, however, some provocative suggestions. Gay and bisexual males with AIDS, it appears, do have access to social support —but in many cases from friends rather than kin. The probability of available informal support appears to be contingent on the existence of identifiable sub-communities of homosexuals or IV drug users; hence it is not at all clear what one should expect regarding the mobilization of social support of homosexuals in nonurban locations where rates of infection are low.

Consequently, an opportunity exists to generate information about age and AIDS and about social support mobilization in the gay and bisexual community, which has implications for understanding aging processes and long-term care in later life. For very old and very dependent persons, mobilizing necessary informal social support from kin alone is not always a realistic possibility. We suggest that gay and bisexual communities, particularly in their response to extraordinarily dependent AIDS patients, will permit an exploration of the dynamics and the limits of mobilizing and sustaining social support systems on a basis other than the implied obligations of kinship. Whether informal social support can be mobilized and sustained for highly dependent, socially stigmatized individuals who cannot rely on the obligations of kinship is a neglected research topic. The study of responses to persons with AIDS will contribute to understanding of long-term care options for older people. An important comparison may be the differential probability of support in urban centers in contrast to small towns and rural areas.

THE SOCIAL EMBEDDEDNESS OF HEALTH AND DISEASE

Societal response to AIDS, both among scientists and laypersons, is an occasion to relearn some old but easily forgotten lessons. The societal allocation of material and social resources is related in complex ways to the risk of disease generally and to particular diseases. The epidemiology of AIDS documents convincingly that the risk of AIDS, at least in early stages of the epidemic, has tended to be heavily concentrated in subpopulations characterized by an unconventional or disadvantaged life-style. As a consequence, societal response to AIDS has been significantly and negatively affected in a variety of ways: by tardy response to the evidence of an epidemic, misinformed fear of contact with AIDS patients, and publicly stated reluctance to allocate societal resources to programs of prevention and treatment of AIDS.

It is not clear from available evidence whether the response of the scientific and lay communities in the United States to AIDS is distinctive or peculiar. Our search of the literature provided no comparative analysis of societal differences in perceptions of or response to the risk of AIDS or to persons with AIDS. Comparative analysis has focused, if at all, on cross-national incidence and prevalence of seropositivity and AIDS cases. We attach some significance, however, to our impression from a systematic search of journal articles on AIDS in Europe and to references to cross-national comparisons in articles published in this country (e.g., Acheson, 1986). The impression is that the visibility of AIDS in the scientific and popular press in the United States is distinctively high. A plausible explanation for a peculiar interest is suggested by the extraordinary ambivalence that is evoked by a life-threatening but poorly understood disease whose most visible victims engaged in life-styles regarded by some as "reprehensible" or "immoral." We would not expect to find a best-selling publication documenting extraordinary widespread ambivalence toward AIDS and persons with AIDS like Randy Shilts's *And the Band Played On* (1987) outside the United States.

Ultimately, we can depend on epidemiologists to provide cross-national evidence on the differential distribution of risk and cases of AIDS in various societies. In the meantime, the usefulness of comparative psychosocial and sociocultural research on perceptions of and responses to AIDS cross-nationally requires no debate. Differential sexual practices in various societies appear to predict differential risk of AIDS. The effects of differential perception of male homosexuality as "just another life-style" or "an abhorrent, tabooed life-style" on whether and how a society proposes to undertake programs of prevention or provide appropriate treatment for AIDS patients are speculative, not definitively documented. We suspect, however, that the dominant sentiments of opinion leaders in a society make a difference in how a society responds in terms of resource mobilization. A related issue is whether and how different societal arrangements for organizing and financing health care affects access to, the effectiveness of, and the cost of health care for persons with AIDS. We suspect also that cross-national research will illustrate that the relatively privatized, fragmented, fee-for-service health care system of the United States is relatively ineffective and inefficient in responding to a devastating chronic illness such as AIDS.

It is worth noting here that even the willingness of our society—perhaps better, governmental resource allocators—to commit resources for research on and treatment of AIDS illustrates the relevance of conflicting societal values in the response to social problems. AIDS, like syphilis a century ago, confronts very basic moral attitudes about sexuality and elicits responses to individuals whose nonnormative sexual preferences place them at risk for a poorly understood and threatening disease. The potential for punitive attitudes and behavior on the part of laypersons would seem obvious enough and could be anticipated. It is less clear whether we should have anticipated the apparent ambivalence of the scientific community about recommending early and urgently that attention and resources should be directed to AIDS. Sociologists of science will eventually find, we argue, that the scientific community's response to AIDS is another illustration of how scientists often remain laypersons insofar as they can and do share general societal values, compete for scientific resources, and on occasion permit their scientific attention to be purchased by the availability of resources for research.

We have also been intrigued by the ways in which weak data have been used both by scientists and laypersons as weapons in support of ideological positions. This is a familiar phenomenon to sociologists, who are sensitive to the uses and abuses of power in human interaction. Rules of social conduct are demonstrably used as weapons for strategic purposes. So also is scientific evidence. In this context, current experience with AIDS will provide an opportunity for future social historians and historians of medicine to demonstrate the usefulness of biomedical models as they relate to the societal embeddedness of conceptions of well-being and how to promote health and prevent or minimize the effects of disease.

CONTRIBUTIONS OF SOCIAL SCIENCE

Overall, in the literature on human aging one is impressed by the substantial proportion of publications that document behavioral and social scientific evidence of the heterogeneity of aging processes, individual differences in aging, and the importance of sociocultural factors in understanding the observed heterogeneity. On the whole, the current literature on AIDS stands in sharp contrast. However, exceptions are beginning to appear in the growing awareness that, if a "silver bullet" solution to AIDS is not an immediate prospect, the only identifiable options in the meantime lie in modifications of individual sexual behaviors, primarily through motivating risk-reducing actions (Fineberg, 1988). The possibility of social control procedures such as mandatory testing and quarantine has continued to receive such a bad press and to activate such concerns about civil liberties that coercive social measures have been minimal.

Significantly, however, in current discussions of the need for financial support of research on AIDS, most proposed agendas do not include a clear mandate for basic behavioral and social scientific research. In general, many allocators of research dollars appear to assume that essential basic behavioral and social scientific research is, in fact, covered by epidemiologic research, or by applied research on interventions designed to modify the behavior of at-risk populations.

Heterogeneity of risk for morbidity, disability, and mortality in later years, however, calls for basic research. It is not simply a matter of charting genes and disease processes. Societies are, in fact, natural experiments in the way in which the allocation of both material (e.g., money and health care) and social (e.g., attitudes, roles, status, education) resources affect aging and the experience of aging. The same logic, we argue, suggests why the behavioral and social sciences will make an important contribution to our understanding of who is at risk for AIDS and why, if we are clever enough, we will eventually conclude that an important form of protection from AIDS will be the reduction of risky individual and social behaviors. Certainly, the history of sexually transmitted diseases, which in the past decade have exhibited increased rates, provides the sobering suggestion that the combination of toxic agents and transmission of these agents by sexual behavior demonstrate the inadequacy of reductionist biomedical models of prevention and cure (Brandt, 1988; Metropolitan Life, 1986; Willis, 1986).

The study of AIDS in an aging society, then, requires recognition of the complementarity of psychosocial and biomedical perspectives in understanding the etiology, course, treatment, and, ultimately, the prevention of AIDS. Only through the utilization of a multidisciplinary approach can we come to understand the disease and the total context in which it develops. The historical trends found in the investigation and treatment of other communicable diseases and the contemporary scientific and health care environments can both be appropriately utilized in the study of the AIDS epidemic. Finally, as we prepare for the future of persons with AIDS and the social environment in which they will live, it is recognition of the relevance of a life-course perspective and the phenomena of aging that can give vital insight into our investigations, projections, interventions, preventions, and care.

REFERENCES

Acheson, D. 1986. "AIDS in the United Kingdom." In *AIDS: An International Forum,* edited by R. Hummel, W. Leavy, M. Rompolla, and S. Chorost. New York: Plenum.

Booth, W. 1988. "CDC Paints a Picture of HIV Infection in the US." *Science* 239:253.

Brandt, A. 1985. *No Silver Bullet: A Social History of Venereal Disease in the United States Since 1880.* New York: Oxford University Press.

———. 1988. "The Syphilis Epidemic and Its Relationship to AIDS." *Science* 239:375–380.

Cohen, S., and L. Syme. (eds.) 1985. *Social Support and Health.* New York: Academic Press.

Curran, J., A. Jaffe, A. Hardy, W. Morgan, R. Selik, and T. Dondero. 1988. "Epidemiology of HIV Infection in the United States." *Science* 239:610–616.

Felman, D., and T. Johnson. (eds.) 1986. *The Social Dimensions of AIDS.* New York: Praeger.

Fineberg, H. 1988. "Education to Prevent AIDS: Prospects and Obstacles." *Science* 239:592–596.

House, J.S., K.R. Landis, and D. Umberson. 1988. "Social Relationships and Health." *Science* 241:540–545.

Institute of Medicine. 1986. *Confronting AIDS: Directions for Public Health, Health Care, and Research.* Washington, DC: National Academy Press.

———. 1988. *Confronting AIDS: Update, 1988.* Washington, DC: National Academy Press.

Janes, C., ed. 1986. *Anthropology and Epidemiology.* New York: Reidel Publishing Co.

Kulstad, R. 1986. *AIDS: Papers from Science: 1982–1985.* Washington, DC: The American Association for the Advancement of Science.

Lambert, B. 1987. "AIDS Forecasts Are Grim—and Disparate." *New York Times* October 25, p. E24.

McKinlay, J., S. McKinlay, and R. Beaglehole. 1988. "Trends in Death and Disease and the Contribution of Medical Measures." In *Handbook of Medical Sociology,* edited by H.E. Freeman and S. Levine. Englewood Cliffs, New Jersey: Prentice-Hall.

Medly, G. et al. 1987. "Incubation Periods of AIDS in Patients via Blood Transfusions." *Nature* 328:719–721.

Metropolitan Life. 1986. "Sexually Transmitted Diseases in the United States." *Statistical Bulletin* 67:3–10.

New England Journal of Medicine. 1987. *AIDS: Epidemiological and Clinical Studies.* Boston: Massachusetts Medical Society.

Osborn, June. 1988. "AIDS: Politics and Science." *New England Journal of Medicine* 318:444–447.

Panem, Sandra. 1988. "Review of And the Band Played On." *Science* 239:1039–1040.

Quinn, T. et al. 1988. "Human Immunodeficiency Virus Infection among Patients Attending Clinics for Sexually Transmitted Diseases." *New England Journal of Medicine* 318:197–203.

Shilts, R. 1987. *And the Band Played On: Politics, People, and the AIDS Epidemic.* New York: St. Martin's Press.

Willis, D. 1986. "AIDS: The Public Context of an Epidemic." *The Milbank Quarterly* 64: Supplement 1 (whole issue).

PART II

Risk Factors and Prevention

CHAPTER 3

A Review of Research on Sexual and AIDS-Related Attitudes and Behaviors

Judith A. Levy and Gary L. Albrecht

Human sexuality is one of the more neglected areas of social research. The lack of information about sexual behavior in the United States has been called "a national embarrassment" (Booth, 1988). This embarrassment has become particularly salient in light of the current AIDS crisis. Ignorance of human sexuality, including the range and frequency of common sexual practices, has hindered attempts to reduce the spread of the disease.

Solid information about the sexual behavior of older adults is particularly scarce. Several factors account for this scarcity. First, commonly accepted norms and beliefs about aging maintain that people past age 60, even past age 50, no longer have interest or engage in sexual behavior. Second, scientific disinterest in human sexuality among older people appears to be tied to demographic factors (Weg, 1983): it is only recently that the large and growing proportion of people living into old age has come to full scientific attention. Third, the sampling and other methodological difficulties inherent in sex research, combined with those encountered in studying older people, have tended to discourage investigators (see Chapter 6 of this volume). Finally, the cost of gathering these data often is considered disproportionately high for the amount of information gained.

Because of the urgent need to deepen understanding of older people's knowledge, attitudes, behavior, and experiences as they relate to both sexuality and AIDS, this chapter reviews key aspects of the relevant literature, thus providing a setting for more specific treatments throughout. It must be emphasized at the

---

The authors received support from the National Institute on Aging for this chapter. They wish to thank Matilda White Riley, Marcia Ory, Diane Zablotsky, and the members of the NIA AIDS Advisory Group for their comments on this work.

outset that the studies covered in the review are necessarily highly selected, and that any review as of 1988 can certainly not keep pace with the continuing barrage of reports on this rapidly changing epidemic.

Several points emerging from this review emphasize the need for a continuing research agenda. In particular, although sexual behavior is a fundamental human activity, little is known of the details of sexuality in late adulthood. Moreover, the number of older people affected by the HIV virus is expected to increase, yet few studies consider how the biological, psychological, and social processes of aging affect transmission and prevention of the disease. Little attention has been paid to unwarranted fears of contracting AIDS, or to how such fears can interfere with the quality of life and can lead to worry and withdrawal from satisfying activities and relationships at any age. In addition, although parents and older family members of people with AIDS are socially, emotionally, and practically affected by this illness, their involvement is largely invisible in the AIDS literature.

In reviewing the literature on such issues, the chapter is divided into five sections. Each takes special note of emphases (or lack of emphases) on the middle and later years of the life course. Studies of sexual attitudes and behaviors are reported in the first section; those of AIDS-related attitudes and behaviors in the second. Within the framework of these first sections, the third section selects for special attention investigations of gay and bisexual males. The fourth section discusses the widespread neglect in much of this literature of middle-aged and older people, noting implications of this neglect. The final section summarizes gaps identified in this literature review, as these gaps contribute to the formulation of a future agenda for research.

SEXUAL ATTITUDES AND BEHAVIORS

Alfred Kinsey's pioneer research (Kinsey, Pomeroy, & Martin, 1948; Kinsey, Pomeroy, Martin, & Gebhard, 1953) on sexual behavior in the human male and female provided the American public with its first documented look at this topic. The Kinsey reports detailed the prevalence and orgasmic frequency of a wide range of sexual behaviors, providing a glimpse into American sexuality that shocked clinicians, scientists, and laymen alike (Weg, 1983). Homosexuality proved far more common than previously suspected, and the range and extent of reported sexual behavior in general questioned existing assumptions about American sexual mores. Despite a massive sample of 18,000 adults, however, the generalizability of Kinsey's findings was limited. The study drew on volunteers, rather than using probability samples, and all participants were white and middle-class. Data collection procedures contained a strong age bias, as older people were not administered the entire instrument and toward the end of the field work were excluded altogether. The final analysis contains information on only 126 males and 56 females over the age of 60. Out of 1,649 pages in the two Kinsey volumes, only four are devoted to older women and three to older men (Starr, 1985).

In an attempt to correct this last deficiency, Christenson and Gagnon (1965) used the noninstitutionalized portion of the case history files of the Institute for Sex Research to analyze face-to-face interviews with a nonrepresentative sample of 241 white females aged 50 through 70. To qualify for inclusion in the sample, respondents had to have been married at least once, but one third were widowed, separated, or divorced at the time they were interviewed. Information obtained through the interviews included the incidence, frequencies, and attitudes of the women toward sex in six areas of sexual behavior: coitus, petting, masturbation, nocturnal sex dreams, homosexual contacts, and contacts with animals. Data were also gathered on the women's sexual anatomy, history of psychosexual arousal, and prepubertal experiences.

Findings from this analysis indicated that these women enjoyed and responded to sexual stimuli throughout their later years, although rates of intercourse, masturbation, and sex dreams gradually diminished with age. Marital coitus was the primary sexual activity for married women at age 50. By age 55, however, frequency of intercourse was lower, but the percentage experiencing coitus remained virtually the same. Masturbation appeared the primary sexual activity for currently unmarried women, and having a sexually active partner strongly influenced both the married and unmarried women's incidence and frequency of coital relations.

Using Kinsey data, Downey (1980) explored male sexuality by attempting to compare the types and frequency of sexual activity for five cohorts of men. Results showed that men born more recently were more likely to have extramarital contacts than those born at an earlier time. Being born in the twentieth century, in contrast to pre-1900, was also associated with reporting a wider range of sexual behavior. Masturbation was reported more frequently among older men who had been born earlier, while nocturnal emissions and homosexual contacts were more common in younger men who were born more recently. This interpretation in terms of cohort differences is suggestive, since cultural changes over the century have undoubtedly affected life-course patterns of sexual behavior. However, given the methodological limitations of the Kinsey research design, it is difficult to separate cohort differences from differences due to aging.

Booth (1988) reports an intriguing story in *Science* about a more recent and potentially rich set of data on sexual behavior that has until recently been withheld from the public. In 1970, the Kinsey Institute contracted with the National Opinion Research Center at the University of Chicago to conduct a national survey of the sexual attitudes and practices of 3,018 randomly selected adults. The survey consisted of two parts. First, face-to-face interviews questioned respondents about their attitudes toward sex. Next, respondents were given a 12-page questionnaire to be filled out in private requesting information on their sexual practices. To gain their confidence and encourage truthfulness, respondents were instructed to return these forms to the investigators in sealed envelopes. After the data were analyzed, however, a dispute over authorship caused a long delay in publication. The data as subsequently released constituted a valuable source of baseline information on changing sexual norms and practices, with applicability to the spread of AIDS.

Masters and Johnson (1966, 1970) added a new methodological dimension to the study of human sexuality by taking their research interests into the laboratory. Initially, using prostitutes and later volunteers, they studied the physiological responses of the body in various states of sexual stimulation and arousal. In addition to contributing to the development of new therapies for sexual dysfunction, their work also exploded a number of popular myths, including the Freudian belief in the vaginal orgasm (Koedt, 1970). The study results, however, have limited generalizability to older people. Of the 694 subjects in the original study, only 20 men and 11 women were older than age 60. Masters and Johnson also used a definition of old age that appears exceedingly youthful by 1980s standards—as beginning at age 40 for women and 50 for men (Starr, 1985)—that is no longer appropriate for research.

Because cross-sectional data like those of Masters and Johnson and—even though he used retrospective questioning—of Kinsey are limited in describing how individuals change their sexual patterns as they grow older, there is a premium on collecting longitudinal data. With this benefit in mind, researchers at the Duke Center for the Study of Aging and Human Development conducted the first Duke Longitudinal Study. They collected medical histories, including sexual behavior, from a sample of 260 volunteers drawn from the nearby community. Collection of the data began in 1954 and continued at two- and three-year intervals for a total of four data points. Interviewers asked respondents about their past and current sexual enjoyment and feelings, their present frequency of intercourse, whether or not intercourse had stopped, and the reasons why.

Findings reported from the first three measurement periods showed one portion of the sample remaining sexually interested and active with advanced age, while another portion gradually lost interest and discontinued sexual activity (Pfeiffer, Verwoerdt, & Wang, 1968). Death of a spouse was the most common reason given by both sexes for discontinuing coitus. The average age for stopping intercourse was 68 for men and 60 for women. By the fourth measurement point, attrition due to death or withdrawal from the study had reduced the original sample from 260 to only 39 people (Pfeiffer, Verwoerdt, & Wang, 1969). But suggestive clues were drawn from this "biologically-advantaged group of aged individuals," as the research team called them. Men continued to report high sexual interest, although the proportion reporting sexual activity declined. Meanwhile, the decline in sexual interest or activity reported by women at phase three showed no further change at this fourth measurement point. Pfeiffer and his colleagues speculate that the lower interest and activity of older women observed in this sample can perhaps be explained by one or more of the following factors: women may undergo declines similar to those of men but at an earlier age; women may have a lower level of sexual interest at all stages of the life course; or the loss of reproductive capacity, associated with a clearly demarcated climacteric, may produce negative psychological feelings toward sex. However, such factors (particularly the last) are hotly debated in the literature and require much further study.

A second Duke Longitudinal Study included data that allowed Pfeiffer and Davis (1972) to explore whether or not male–female differences in reported sexual behavior in old age may have their antecedents in middle age. Subjects for the analysis were 502 people between 45 and 69 years of age who had been randomly selected from the lists of a local medical plan. The questions on sexual behavior focused on respondents' enjoyment, frequency, and any possible decline of sexual functioning. Findings indicate that past sexual enjoyment, marital status, and age best predict continued interest and sexual behavior among women. A far larger number of variables predict sexual interest and behavior in men. Understandably, having a sexually capable partner affects coital relations for both sexes, although the greater longevity of women, coupled with societal disapproval of extramarital relations, meant that this association was stronger for women than for men.

Other studies also have considered how gender roles and sex differences influence sexual behavior. Hite (1976, 1978), for example, polled the readers of large circulation, popular magazines in an attempt to determine differences in male and female sexual needs and desires. Hite's findings, though controversial, indicated that most American women were dissatisfied with the standard amount of foreplay preceding sexual intercourse, and a greater proportion of women than men reported chronic sexual dissatisfaction with coital relations. Men, by contrast, complained that women were less interested in sex than males, rarely made sexual advances toward their partners, and typically assumed a passive role during sexual relations. Hite's study has been strongly criticized on methodological grounds, including the biases introduced by using a self-selected sample (Heiman, 1978). A study of college men and women, however, does support Hite's findings that women appear to derive more pleasure from foreplay and afterplay than men, while men find comparatively greater enjoyment in the act of sexual intercourse (Denny, Field, & Quadagno, 1984).

In sum, a review of selected major studies of human sexuality over the last 40 years suggests that sexual interest and activity continue into old age, although there is a decline in frequency and type for most, but not all, elderly adults (Starr, 1985). Men and women tend to differ in interest and activity, but the reasons for these differences are unclear.

Meanwhile, a review of the methods used in these studies emphasizes the limitations of the findings. Practically all, with the notable exception of Masters and Johnson (1966, 1970), are based on self-reported data, a condition that raises serious questions about the truthfulness and accuracy of respondents' reports. Generalizability of the findings is limited as, with few exceptions, researchers rely on volunteers rather than probability samples, and these samples are too often comprised exclusively of white, middle-class participants. Age is poorly represented as a variable: most samples fall within the age range of 18 to 50, with few older people included. Typically, the data collected consist of "counts" of the frequency and type of homosexual or heterosexual behavior in which people engage. Sexuality is implicitly conceptualized either as a solitary pursuit, involving masturbation, or as a purely physiological exchange between two people, rather than as social interaction. Although Schur (1988) convincingly argues that cultural priorities and social relationships organize sexuality, there are few studies that examine sex behavior as a social activity. Indeed, scientific concern about the social processes and consequences of human sexuality appear to have remained dormant until the spread of life-threatening sexually-transmitted diseases (STDs) such as AIDS and the reemergence of syphilis pressured the scientific community for information and answers.

AIDS-RELATED ATTITUDES AND BEHAVIORS

While our review of research on sexual attitudes and behaviors begins four decades ago, our review of research on AIDS covers less than a single decade. The AIDS "crisis," along with concern about the spread of other serious sexually transmitted diseases, sparked increased interest in sexual research and, perhaps, added to its respectability as a topic of scientific inquiry.

Studies of Age-Related Attitudes

Much of the earliest information on the general public's attitudes, knowledge, and behavior about AIDS was collected through public opinion polls conducted by major newspapers, the national broadcasting networks, and polling organizations (Singer, Rogers, & Corcoran, 1987). Early polls include Gallup (June, 1983; July, 1983; June, 1985; August 1985; November, 1985; April, 1986), the Los Angeles *Times* (December, 1985), the National Broadcasting Company (NBC) and *The Wall Street Journal* (November 1985; January, 1986), and the American Broadcasting Company (ABC) and the *Washington Post* (September 1985; September, 1985).

Survey questions about AIDS have differed by poll, although the items cover a wide range of topics when viewed as a set. General areas of inquiry include public knowledge about transmission of the HIV virus, attitudes toward people with AIDS, opinions on issues of public policy, and personal fear of AIDS. The polls often handle sensitive questions about sexual and AIDS high-risk behavior through projective questions that ask respondents to comment on other people's practices rather than their own. With the exception of Gallup, polls rarely report their results by age categories. According to the Gallup Poll for April 1986, for example, people over 65 are somewhat more likely than younger people to say they have not heard about AIDS, or that they believe the virus is transmitted through casual contact.

The National Center for Health Statistics began in August 1987 to include in the National Health Interview Survey (NHIS) questions about the adult population's knowledge, attitude, and behavior toward AIDS. The added items are designed to provide baseline information and to allow measurement of changes over time. Results are reported by three age categories: 18 to 29, 30 to 49, and 50 and older. Results for the first month of data collection indicate substantial differences by age (National Center for Health Statistics, 1987). Adults over the age of 50 are more likely than younger people to state that they "know nothing" about AIDS, and fewer older people than young reported knowing "a lot." People over 50 were also somewhat more likely than younger people to perceive that AIDS could be transmitted through casual contact (such as eating in restaurants where the cook has AIDS; sharing food implements; working near or kissing someone who has the disease; or using public toilets). Conversely, people over 50 were less likely than the younger segments of the sample to associate the transmission of the AIDS virus with the practice of sharing needles during illegal drug use. They were less likely to have heard of the blood test for HIV-specific antibodies or to indicate willingness to be tested. Moreover, they appeared less well informed about the efficacy of various prophylactics, including condoms, in preventing transmission of the virus.

Studies of AIDS-Related Behavior

Albrecht, Levy, and Sugrue (1987) conducted one of the first studies of the knowledge, attitudes, and behavior of the general public toward AIDS that also included specific questions about intimate sexual behavior. The research, supported in part by the Centers for Disease Control (CDC), was conducted during 1986–1987 through the Comprehensive AIDS Prevention/Education Program at the City of Chicago Department of Health and by the University of Illinois at Chicago. Telephone interviews were made with 1,540 adults between the ages of 18 and 60 residing in households in Chicago and the surrounding suburban area, using random digit dialing to include unlisted numbers (see Blair & Czaja, 1982; Waksberg, 1978). Because both groups are at high risk, blacks and Hispanics were oversampled. Although people over 60 were not included in the sample, 35% of the respondents were between 18 and 29, 35% between 30 and 39, and 30% between 40 and 60. Preliminary findings indicate, for example, that low education and being Hispanic predict never having heard of AIDS, but no significant age differences were found in the probability of having heard about the disease (Albrecht et al., 1988). Moreover, people between the ages of 40 and 60, when compared to younger people in the sample, are less likely to perceive themselves at risk for AIDS, or to report having modified their behavior to avoid risk. They also are somewhat less likely to have had vaginal or anal intercourse in the past 5 years, and they report fewer current partners.

Several other general population studies of AIDS and sexual behavior have been instituted since the Albrecht et al. data were collected. One of the more controversial studies is that by Masters, Johnson, and Kolodny (1988), *CRISIS: Heterosexual Behavior in the Age of AIDS.* The highly specialized sample of 800 men and women between the ages of 21 and 40 was recruited from churches, singles bars, and colleges in New York City, Atlanta, and St. Louis. This sample was designed to allow comparison of the sexual habits and presence of the virus in two extreme categories of sexually active people: those who are monogamous and those with at least six heterosexual partners each year. The investigators report that, of the 400 people who had been monogamous for the past 5 years, only one tested positive for HIV antibodies. Of the comparison sample reporting at least six partners a year, however, 6% were found to be infected. The research design and many of the assertions made in the book have been strongly criticized on methodological grounds by health experts, including U.S. Surgeon General C. Everett Koop and Stephen Joseph, the Health Commissioner for New York City, where a portion of the data were collected. Among Masters et al.'s assertions: The virus is spreading to the heterosexual population of the United States at rates twice as high as official estimates; transmission of the virus can in principle occur through contact with virus-contaminated articles such as toothbrushes and toilet seats. Critics averred that no corroborative scientific evidence for such assertions currently exists.

In 1988, for the first time, the National Opinion Research Center (NORC) at the University of Chicago included in the long-established General Social

Survey items about sexual behavior and AIDS. The questions about AIDS, which are interviewer-administered, ask for opinions on political, educational, and public health issues, and also for attitudes toward people with AIDS. Respondents are asked to indicate the number of people (living or dead) that they have known with the disease; their relationship to the one person with AIDS best known to them; and that person's sex, age, race, and current morbidity/mortality status. The more personal sexual questions (some of which are self-administered in the presence of the interviewer) ask respondents to report their total number of sexual partners in the past 12 months, the gender of these partners, and their relationship to the respondent. Data from the General Social Survey are widely used for analysis by private subscribers and through the data repositories of most major universities.

Currently under way at the National Opinion Research Center (NORC) at the University of Chicago, with Edward Laumann as Principal Investigator, is a project for designing a survey of sexual practices, AIDS, and health in the general population.[1] This effort involved a review of the literature on sexual practices, sexually transmitted diseases, and fertility-related behavior as a basis for development and pretesting of instruments. At the time of this writing, plans included an interview schedule consisting of a 45-minute core questionnaire concerning sexual attitudes and behavior. In addition, respondents were to be given a self-administered questionnaire to be filled out in private and returned in a sealed envelope to the research team. An interesting feature of the design is its use of the life-course perspective. This perspective is considered appropriate as it permits biological maturation and physiological age markers and events to be combined with age norms and social life events in predicting and understanding the sequence, timing, and duration of human sexual behavior. In addition, the aim was to focus on the sexual dyad as the basic social unit in which sex occurs and through which disease is spread. Thus, data will be collected using a social network framework.

International Studies

Broadening the framework of research that is conducted exclusively in the United States, the World Health Organization's Special Programme on the Social and Behavioral Aspects of AIDS, under the directorship of Dr. Manuel Carballo, has been designing a 35- to 50-nation survey of people's knowledge, attitudes, beliefs, and high-risk practices in relation to AIDS. With such information, the World Health Organization and the health ministries of the

[1] This section profited from the incisive and detailed discussion of network analysis and the life-course perspective applied to the study of human sexual behavior in the technical proposal of the National Opinion Research Center, "Social and Behavioral Aspects of Health and Fertility Related Behavior."

individual countries can mount targeted educational and risk intervention programs suited to the needs of specific populations, and they can use subsequent surveys to ascertain the impact of AIDS on the lives of individuals. The plan included three interrelated surveys, to be conducted in each country: (1) a general population survey of adults; (2) a survey of health care workers, especially those who have contact with persons with AIDS; and (3) a survey of health policy makers to ascertain their knowledge, perceptions, actions, and resources devoted to the problem. Added modules can deal with special topics pertinent to individual countries. Special attention was given here to the problems of interviewing illiterate people, individuals in different cultures and subcultures, and the different contexts and interpretations of AIDS in local settings. For example, AIDS in Africa is transmitted heterosexually and through an unmonitored black market blood supply. In certain countries, AIDS is perceived by some to be a result of a curse or witchcraft rather than high-risk sexual behavior.

In another set of multinational general population surveys, Gail Wilensky and the staff at The Center for Health Affairs, Project Hope, have been working with Louis Harris Associates to evaluate the impact of major AIDS educational/risk reduction strategies on individual risk-related behaviors. These initial surveys were conducted in France, Great Britain, and the United States during the summer of 1988. These countries were suitable for the first phase of the study because they had all instituted major AIDS education/risk reduction programs and their populations could be surveyed easily. A core questionnaire allowed data to be compared within and between countries. The further evaluation will use both questionnaire and reported health statistics in a time series design to measure the effects of the interventions.

Other Intervention Studies

As another example of an intervention project, CDC has funded a one-year demonstration project at the University of Illinois School of Public Health, with Wayne W. Wiebel as Principal Investigator. The aim is to reduce the spread of AIDS among Chicago IV drug users, their sexual partners, and prostitutes associated with IV drug use. The project uses a team intervention model to dispense written materials about AIDS prevention and to teach IV drug users and their sexual partners how to avoid infection. Each team is comprised of a seasoned ethnographer and two indigenous health workers who are themselves former drug users who have completed a methadone treatment program. The health workers are given extensive training in information about AIDS and the HIV virus, then sent into the "shooting galleries" in three city locations where drugs are sold. Their job includes dispensing written materials about AIDS, teaching addicts to clean their needles, and encouraging safer drug-use habits. The overall mission of the study includes outreach to targeted populations; interagency coordination to assist in achieving demonstration objectives; referral for drug abuse treatment and other service needs; AIDS prevention/education; promotion of risk reduction; and research evaluation.

SEX AND AIDS IN GAY POPULATIONS

The early spread of AIDS in the gay community, and the predominance of gay and bisexual men as a source for transmission of the disease, has produced a body of research especially focused on gay populations. (Compare the chapters in this volume by Stall, Catania, and Pollack and by Catania et al.) Most of the studies of gay populations and AIDS are designed to investigate frequency of sexual behavior associated with transmission of the virus and gay males' response to the threat of developing the disease. A few of the studies of gay men examine age as a factor. Studies of gay women and AIDS are largely absent from the literature, perhaps because lesbians have been at comparatively low risk for the disease.

Sexual and AIDS-Related Attitudes and Behaviors

In 1987, in order to find out what is scientifically known about older gay men, Lee searched the literature for homosexual aspects of aging. His review included studies with at least one or two questions on sexual attraction, age, and type of preferred partners (Bell & Weinberg, 1978). Also included were studies of homosexual practices and fantasies (Humphreys, 1970; Kelly, 1977; Lee, 1978; Lehne, 1974).

An early study that shows age differences in gay men's response to AIDS was conducted by the San Francisco AIDS Foundation (Bye, 1984, 1985). A probability sample was obtained through a telephone screening of the general population, in contrast to the more usual recruitment through bars, newspaper advertisements, street intercepts, and organizational referrals. The study design consisted of a two-wave telephone survey of the sexual behavior and knowledge about AIDS of 500 self-identified gay and bisexual male residents of San Francisco, California. All respondents were at least 18 years of age; almost half were in their thirties; one third were age 40 or more; and only 2% were over age 65. Although the study reported few findings specifically related to the later years, a strong linear relationship was found between age and having a primary relationship with a male partner. Older men appeared less likely to be in primary relationships than younger men, a finding substantiated in an earlier study by Weinberg and Williams (1974). Respondents over 45 also were less likely to report using "safe sex" measures. Phase two of the study, conducted in 1985, confirms the previous year's findings and lends further support to other studies that show a decline in the frequency of "at risk" sexual acts and number of partners among gay men. (For another review of this study, see the chapter in this volume by Catania et al.)

Changing Life-Styles of Gay Men

The accumulating evidence suggests that many gay men are changing their life-styles in response to perceived risk of AIDS. For example, McKusick, Horstman, and Coates (1985) report that sexual activity in a sample of 655 gay men in San Francisco declined over a one-year period between 1982 and 1983. The gay men reported less use of bathhouses for sexual encounters; fewer engaged in "unsafe sex" practices such as anal intercourse; and the number of men who reported five or more sexual partners decreased over that time period. Similar results have been reported among gay men in New York (Feldman, 1986; Martin, 1987; Stall et al., 1986), Wisconsin (Golubjatnikov, Pfister, & Tillotson, 1983), and Chicago (Emmons et al., 1986; Joseph et al., 1987). See Becker and Joseph (1988) for an excellent review of this body of research.

Barriers to sexual change among gay men have also been investigated. For example, the Multicenter AIDS Cohort Study in Chicago, funded by the National Institute of Allergy and Infectious Diseases, was designed to assess the biomedical natural history of AIDS among gay men (Emmons et al., 1986). The sample was primarily white (91.1%) and had a mean age of 34.6 years, an average of 16.2 years of education, and 16.5 years of homosexual experience. Respondents were generally found to believe that behavioral changes could reduce their risk of contracting the virus. Actual behavior change, however, was linked to belief in the future ability of biomedical technology to prevent or cure AIDS, the perceived pressure of social norms, and perceived difficulties in controlling one's sexual impulses. No significant relationship was found between a measure of gay social network affiliations and behavioral outcome. Analyses by age were not reported.

THE NEGLECTED ROLE OF OLDER ADULTS

Throughout this review, the paucity of current and projected future information on sexuality, AIDS, and aging leads to an important question: What is known about sex and AIDS in relation to older adults? Further examination of the literature, with reference to the various sources of transmission, shows that, at least through 1987, young and middle-aged people in the United States are far more likely than older people to be infected with the HIV virus or to develop AIDS. Nonetheless, incidence rates presented in the chapter by Stall, Catania, and Pollack in this volume indicate that people aged 50 and older made up approximately 10% of the total number of cases each year between 1982 and 1987. Should this age distribution hold, Moss and Miles (1987) project that over 27,000 AIDS cases by 1991 will be in persons over age 50. Of these, 1,100 will be people over 70 years old.

It is difficult to know how much confidence to place in these and other projections. (See the chapter in this volume by Manton and Singer.) Estimates of the rate of AIDS transmission differ widely among researchers and some, such as those by Masters, Johnson, and Kolodny (see Grady, 1988; Monmaney, 1988), are hotly disputed. Carne et al. (1987) contend that, for the most part, epidemiologists and other scientists have overestimated the spread of the AIDS virus among young and middle-aged adults. Meanwhile, projections for older people have received scant epidemiological attention or assessment. Clues to the spread of AIDS among older people, however, can be found in studies that compare, within the major categories of transmission, the sexual and life-style patterns of older adults with those of high-risk younger adults.

Homosexual Encounters

Currently the majority of new cases of AIDS in the United States are transmitted through homosexual encounters and are heavily concentrated among men between the ages of 30 and 40 (Stall, Catania, & Pollack, this volume; Selwyn, 1986). Nonetheless, little solid data are available indicating the number of people in the United States who perceive themselves as gay, much less their ages. Thus the denominators are missing for computing incidence *rates* of AIDS among gay men. During the late 1940s, Kinsey and his colleagues (1948) estimated that 10% of American males are more or less exclusively homosexual for a period of at least 3 years between the ages of 16 and 55; 4% were estimated to be homosexual throughout life. The 4% estimate has been replicated in a number of successive studies (Darrow, Gorman, & Glick, 1986), although subpopulation differences may exist. Gagnon and Simon (1973) found slightly lower rates when they reanalyzed these data for a subsample of college men under the age of 30.

Estimates of homosexuality as the base for and the spread of rates of incidence or prevalence of AIDS are sensitive to a number of factors. For example, the gay revolution of the 1960s and 1970s encouraged many gay men and women to be open about their sexual preferences and behavior. Thus, to some extent statistics summarizing homosexual practices before and after this period reflect differences in reporting rather than behavioral change. In addition, young gay men and women tend to migrate to certain urban areas, particularly

New York, Chicago, Houston, Los Angeles, and San Francisco. Homosexuality, relatively youthful populations, and the spread of the AIDS virus all peak in these particular geographic locales. For example, as noted, the recent study by Bye (1984), using local registries and a snowball sample, found that nearly one half of men living in San Francisco who openly identify themselves as gay or bisexual are in their thirties; few are elderly or retired. Nonetheless, this group is expected to increase dramatically as middle-aged men in this population mature and reach retirement age. Accordingly, there is opportunity for the proportion of older men with AIDS to rise also.

In the meantime, today's older gay males may be at less risk for AIDS than their younger counterparts when patterns of life-style are considered. Earlier research notes that men over 45 tend to visit gay establishments comparatively less, are more likely to live alone, and have greater difficulty finding sexual partners (Weinberg & Williams, 1974). Accordingly, they may have less frequent sexual encounters and, perhaps, lower exposure to the HIV virus. Also, while older gay men may have younger sexual partners (Harry & DeVall, 1978), most prefer men their own age (Kelly, 1977)—a preference that may provide some insulation against infection though sexual contact with younger, high-risk males. An exception may involve older, middle-class men who frequent gay bars, as some evidence suggests that they prefer younger partners. In any case, any advantages of older age and the associated life-styles may be offset by the tendency of older gay men to reject using "safe sex" measures (Bye, 1984). In addition, the biological and immunological changes with aging, often accompanied by possible declines in health status, may place older gay men at added risk. Such assumptions need scientific investigation.

Intravenous (IV) Drug Use

After gay men, IV drug abusers are currently the next highest population group at risk for AIDS (except for people 50 and over, cf. Stall, Catania, & Pollack in this volume). Most IV drug abusers are young (Wish, 1987), and nearly 80% of those who acquire AIDS through parenteral transmission are diagnosed before 40 years of age (Allen & Curran, 1988). Women tend to be diagnosed at younger ages than men, which may reflect either different susceptibility to the virus or patterns of drug use. Older adults who are IV drug abusers are reported to be found in geographic areas where low-grade heroine is sold. Because so few illegal drug users are over age 50, parenteral transmission seems unlikely to affect much of the country's older population directly. Perhaps of greater relevance, the HIV virus can also be transmitted through sexual contact with IV drug abusers, or with the sexual partners of IV drug abusers, including prostitutes (Quinn et al., 1988), but no data were found on how many middle-aged or older people either belong to, or engage in sex with, this high-risk group.

Blood-Related Transmission

Since contact with contaminated blood products is another significant means through which the HIV virus is transmitted, hemophiliacs and recipients of blood transfusions are at special risk. (See the chapter by Catania et al. in this volume.) Hemophilia is a hereditary blood-clotting disorder that occurs almost exclusively in males. Most hemophiliacs die by middle adulthood, leaving few at risk for AIDS in old age (Stehr-Green et al., 1988). By contrast, nonhemophiliacs who contract the HIV virus through blood transfusions tend to be older (Curran et al., 1985), and they often have spouses or other sexual partners whom they place at risk (Peterman et al., 1988; Pitchenik et al., 1983, 1984). To be sure, blood-related transmission of AIDS has been reduced considerably by improvements in the production of synthetic blood and by procedures for detecting the HIV antibodies in plasma (Institute of Medicine, National Academy of Science, 1986). Nonetheless, the incubation period for testing seropositive for HIV antibodies is extensive; it has been estimated at about 5.44 years for people over 60 (Medley et al., 1987). Over the next few years, then, new cases of AIDS are expected to develop among older people who had transfusions prior to 1985, when testing procedures first went into effect. Meanwhile, many Third World countries do not screen their blood supplies effectively, and blood is sold on the black market. This situation increases the risk of exposure by U.S. citizens when traveling to countries where these practices are in force.

Heterosexual Transmission

Unlike many Third World countries where this source of transmission predominates, rates of heterosexually acquired AIDS in the United States are low when compared to the proportion of cases attributable to homosexuality and IV drug abuse (see Chapter 4 by Stall, Catania, & Pollack in this volume, Tables 4.2 and 4.3). Allen and Curran (1988) report that females with heterosexually acquired AIDS tend to be younger at diagnosis than females who develop AIDS through parenteral infection or when compared to males in any risk group. (Of females diagnosed with heterosexually acquired AIDS in 1987, 30.9% were less than 30 years of age and 81.3% were under age 40.) Allen and Curran suggest that these age patterns may reflect women's tendency to engage in sexual activity at an earlier age than men, and also to have sex with older men who may be at higher risk for HIV infection. Meanwhile, the incidence of heterosexual transmission in adults over age 50 has risen from 1.3% of the total number of cases in 1982 to 4.6% in 1987 (see Stall, Catania, & Pollack in this volume, Tables 4.3 and 4.4D). This increase contrasts with a trend toward a slight decline in heterosexual transmission for other age groups.

In sum, examination of the literature on existing AIDS rates and transmission routes indicates that older people account for proportionately fewer new cases of AIDS than young and middle-aged adults. Nonetheless, when compared to other means of transmission, the proportion of sexually acquired AIDS cases (both homosexual and heterosexual) as diagnosed in adults over age 50 still occurs at substantially high rates when compared with younger populations. This finding is unexpected given the lower frequency of sexual relations for older populations reported by researchers (Downey, 1980; Pfeiffer et al., 1968; Pfeiffer & Davis, 1972; and more recently in the NORC data from the General Social Survey). Moreover, findings sprinkled throughout the human sexuality literature suggest that cohorts of people now old, who completed puberty and marital courtship prior to the sexual revolution of the 1960s, may perhaps have fewer sexual partners over their lifetime in part because they learned early to subscribe to sexual norms more closely approximating "safe sex" (see Hunt, 1974; Starr & Weiner, 1981). The seeming contradiction between patterns of sexual conduct in later years as reported in the scientific literature and unexpected rates of sexually transmitted disease for the same older population calls attention to the need for research that tests current scientific assumptions, opens new lines of theoretical and factual inquiry, and provides added information and insights about sexual beliefs and behavior in cohorts of people born at different times and across all stages of the life-course, including middle to late adulthood and old age.

NOTES ON AN AGENDA FOR FUTURE RESEARCH

To date, little is known of the sexual knowledge, attitudes, and activity of people at all stages of the life course, but particularly for individuals in late adulthood and old age. In addition, few research findings or theoretical insights are available that examine or explain older adults' beliefs and behaviors toward AIDS or people who have the disease. Yet studies of these concerns within the context of age and aging are critical if we are to gain a better understanding of sexual behavior and its consequences across the human life-course and within specific life transitions and stages.

Human aging entails more than biological change. Clearly it also involves change in psychological processes and in interactive processes of social relationships. As people mature in chronological age, they simultaneously pass through a sequence of interrelated biological and life-course events that shape their sexual development and behavior. The properties and conditions of one stage form the basic starting point for the next. Among older women, for example, ontogenetic processes such as menopause potentially interact with individual life-course events such as widowhood to produce varying patterns of sexual conduct and risk for sexually transmitted disease. Thus life-course studies are needed that identify continuities and discontinuities in sexual patterns, conduct, and risk factors for people of all sexual orientations and age groups, including older adults. Studies of older people seem particularly important because their attitudes and behavior represent the culmination of a lifetime of earlier sexual and life-course experience. From the standpoint of evaluating programs designed to reduce the spread of AIDS, knowledge of the varied patterns of persistence and change in human sexuality across the life course are crucial.

The frequently long period of latency from initial exposure to development of symptoms of AIDS presents another of the more neglected, yet critical, areas of AIDS and aging research. (Compare the chapter by Maddox in this volume.) Models are needed for predicting the numbers of young and middle-aged people who are already exposed to or carrying the virus and who may develop the disease in later life. Exploration is needed of the social, psychological, and ethical difficulties, and the strategies for coping with uncertainty, entailed by testing seropositive for the virus. For example, to what extent, if at all, do older persons who received blood transfusions prior to 1985 worry about developing AIDS? How does the possibility of exposure to the virus affect their marital relationships, including sexual practices? Do postmenopausal couples employ or feel comfortable using condoms to prevent transmission of the virus once the possibility of pregnancy ends?

Although most sexual behavior takes place between two or more actors and within the structure of a social environment, previous studies have focused primarily on isolated individuals. This limitation constrains our ability to model the spread of AIDS, and the variability in life-course patterns as individuals mature. Because such patterns of sexual conduct are embedded in social relationships, the bonds between partners are important foci for analyses of the spread of sexually transmitted disease. The boundaries and permeability of such networks vary widely and are shaped by such influences as the characteristics, preferences, life-style, and social circumstances of the members of whom they are composed. Over the course of a lifetime, individuals are likely to join and withdraw from a number of networks, including those linked by sexual bonds. Thus far, network analysis of human sexuality and its relation to the spread of AIDS has only begun to unravel a few of the many forces and factors that structure these networks and the attitudes and behavior of people within them (see the NORC pilot project cited above).

In terms of preventing transmission of the HIV virus, it also is important to identify how sexual activity across the life-course interacts with associated risk factors to AIDS, such as poor health, substance abuse, and infection with other sexually transmitted diseases (STDs). More studies are needed that focus on the double jeopardy of being at risk simultaneously through sexual behavior and other sources of infection such as IV drug abuse (cf. Stall et al., 1986). Although most attention to the transmission of AIDS has focused on homosexual males or on IV drug abusers, there will be increasing need for knowledge about other groups at risk (heterosexuals, people with hemophilia, and those who receive contaminated blood products during surgery), and about how one route of transmission affects another at varying ages.

Regardless of the mechanism of transmission, AIDS and other STDs are highly stigmatized health conditions. (See the chapter by McKinlay et al. in this volume.) Fear and the negative social judgments that surround these diseases can affect the person's relationships with family members, spouse, and friends. It is important to know where and how older adults receive their general health information and their understandings and beliefs about AIDS. Yet we have little understanding of the extent to which social evaluations of sexual conduct influence people's perception of AIDS and those infected with the virus.

As is true for all age categories, the sexual history and attitudes of older people have important implications for how they view individuals who develop AIDS, including members of their immediate families and social networks. In some instances, older adults may become the caregivers of their children, grandchildren or husbands or wives who develop AIDS. In other instances, as AIDS victims themselves, they may be the recipients of care by others. As more AIDS patients are placed in nursing homes and other health care facilities, it will become increasingly important from a social policy and programmatic standpoint to understand the reactions of older people and their families. Nonetheless, studies of older people's position and participation in networks of support for treatment, care, and prevention of AIDS have been noticeably absent from the literature. (See the chapter in this volume by Crystal.)

Despite these and other reasons for investigating sex and AIDS among older populations, much of the research currently under way still appears to ignore older adults as much as previous research has done. This chapter was written in the hope of encouraging more such investigation through examination and evaluation of the literature that defines the limits, as well as the strengths, of previous research. This literature review calls attention to the many critical issues and research questions that remain. Until more social scientists are willing to tackle the study of sexual conduct among older people, our understanding of sex as a fundamental human process throughout the life course, and its relationship to AIDS as a serious health problem that affects all age groups, will remain scientifically uncharted and potentially misleading.

REFERENCES

Albrecht, G., J. Levy, and N.M. Sugrue. 1987. "Evaluation Component of the City of Chicago's AIDS Risk Reduction/Prevention Program." Project funded 10/1/87–9/30/87 by Centers for Disease Control, U.S. Public Health Service.

Albrecht, G.L., J.A. Levy, N.M. Sugrue, T. Prohaska, and D.G. Ostrow. 1988. "Who Hasn't Heard About AIDS?" Chicago: draft.

Allen, J.R., and J.W. Curran. 1988. "Prevention of AIDs and HIV Infection: Needs, and Priorities for Epidemiologic Research." *The American Journal of Public Health* 78:381–386.

Becker, M.H., and J.G. Joseph. 1988. "AIDS and Behavioral Change to Reduce Risk: A Review." *The American Journal of Public Health* 78:394–410.

Bell, A.P., and M.S. Weinberg. 1978. *Homosexualities.* New York: Simon & Schuster.

Blair, J., and R. Czaja. 1982. "Locating A Special Population Using Random Digit Dialing." *Public Opinion Quarterly* 46:585–590.

Booth, W. 1988. "The Long, Lost Survey on Sex." *Science* 239:1084–1085.

Bye, L. 1984. "Designing An Effective AIDS Prevention Campaign Strategy for San Francisco: Results from the First Probability Sample of An Urban Gay Community." San Francisco, The San Francisco AIDS Foundation.

———. 1985. "Designing An Effective AIDS Prevention Campaign Strategy for San Francisco: Results from a Second Probability Sample of An Urban Gay Community." San Francisco: The San Francisco AIDS Foundation.

Carne, C.A., A.M. Johnson, F. Pearce, A. Smith, R.S. Tedder, I.V. Weller, C. Loveday, A. Hawkins, P. Williams, and M.W. Adler. 1987. "Prevalence of Antibodies to Human Immunodeficiency Virus, Gonorrhoea Rates, and Changed Sexual Behavior in Homosexual Men in London." *The Lancet* 1:656–658.

Christenson, C.V. and J.H. Gagnon. 1965. "Sexual Behavior in a Group of Older Women." *Journal of Gerontology* 20:351–356.

Curran, J.W., N.W. Jaffe, T.A. Peterman, and J.R. Allen. 1985. "Epidemiological Aspects of Acquired Immunodeficiency Syndrome (AIDS) in the United States: Cases Associated with Transfusions." *Progress in Clinical Biological Research* 182:259–269.

Darrow, W.W., E.M. Gorman, and B.P. Glick. 1986. "The Social Origin of AIDS: Social Change, Sexual Behavior and Disease Trends." Pp. 95–107 in *The Social Dimensions of AIDS: Methods and Theory,* edited by D.A. Feldman and T.M. Johnson. New York: Praeger.

Denney, N.W., J.K. Field, and D. Quadagno. 1984. "Sex Differences in Sexual Needs and Desires." *Archives of Sexual Behavior* 13:233–245.

Downey, L. 1980. "Intergenerational Change in Sex Behavior: A Belated Look at Kinsey's Males." *Archives of Sexual Behavior* 9:267–317.

Emmons, C.A., J.G. Joseph, R.C. Kessler, C.B. Wortman, S.B. Montgomery, and D.G. Ostrow. 1986. "Psychosocial Predictors of Reported Behavior Changes in Homosexual Men at Risk for AIDS." *Health Education Quarterly* 13:331–345.

Feldman, D.A. 1986. "AIDS Health Promotion and Clinically Applied Anthropology." In *The Social Dimensions of AIDS: Method and Theory,* edited by D.A. Feldman and T.M. Johnson. New York: Praeger.

Gagnon, J., and W. Simon. 1973. *Sexual Conduct: The Social Sources of Human Sexuality.* Chicago: Aldine.

Golubjatnikov, R., J. Pfister, and T. Tillotson. 1983. "Homosexual Promiscuity and the Fear of AIDS." *Lancet* II:681.

Grady, D. March 21, 1988. "Just How Does AIDS Spread?" *Time,* 60–61.
Harry, J., and W. DeVall. 1978. "Age and Sexual Culture Among Homosexually Oriented Males." *Archives of Sexual Behavior* 7:199–209.
Heiman, J.R. 1978. "Book Review: The Hite Report." *Archives of Sexual Behavior* 7:69–71.
Hite, S. 1976. *The Hite Report: A Nationwide Study of Female Sexuality.* New York: Macmillan.
———. 1978. *The Hite Report on Male Sexuality.* New York: Knopff.
Humphreys, L. 1970. *Tearoom Trade: Impersonal Sex in Public Places* (2nd ed., 1975). Chicago: Aldine.
Hunt, M. 1974. *Sexual Behavior in the 1970s.* Chicago: Playboy Press.
Institute of Medicine, National Academy of Science, Committee on a National Strategy for AIDS. 1986. "Understanding Of The Disease And Dimensions Of The Epidemic." Pp. 37–84 in *Confronting AIDS: Directions for Public Health, Health Care, and Research.* Washington, D.C.: National Academy Press.
Joseph, J.G., S.B. Montgomery, C.A. Emmons, R.C. Kessler, D.G. Ostrow, C.B. Wortman, K. O'Brien, M. Eller, and S. Eshelman. 1987. "Magnitude and Determinants of Behavioral Risk Reduction: Longitudinal Analysis of a Cohort at Risk for AIDS." *Psychological Health* 1:73–96.
Kelly, J. 1977. "The Aging Male Homosexual: Myth and Reality." *The Gerontologist* 17:328–332.
Kinsey, A.C., W.B. Pomeroy, and C.R. Martin. 1948. *Sexual Behavior in the Human Male.* Philadelphia: Sanders.
Kinsey, A.C., W.B. Pomeroy, C.R. Martin, and P. Gebhard. 1953. *Sexual Behavior in the Human Female.* Philadelphia: Saunders.
Koedt, A. 1970. *The Myth of Vaginal Orgasm.* Pittsburgh: Know, Inc.
Lee, J.A. 1978. *Getting Sex.* Toronto: General.
———. 1987. "What Can Homosexual Aging Studies Contribute to Theories of Aging?" *Journal of Homosexuality* 13:43–71.
Lehne, G. 1974. "Gay Male Fantasies." *The Body Politic* Sept.:20–22.
Martin, J.L. 1987. "The Impact of AIDS on Gay Male Sexual Behavior Patterns in New York City." *American Journal of Public Health* 77:578–581.
Masters, W.H., and V.E. Johnson. 1966. *Human Sexual Response.* Boston: Little, Brown.
———. 1970. *Human Sexual Inadequacy.* Boston: Little, Brown.
Masters, W.H., V.E. Johnson, and R.C. Kolodny. 1988. *CRISIS: Heterosexual Behavior in the Age of AIDS.* New York: Grove Press.
McKusick, L., W. Horstman, and T.J. Coates. 1985. "AIDS and Sexual Behavior Reported by Gay Men in San Francisco." *American Journal of Public Health* 75(5):493–496.
Medley, G.F., R.M. Anderson, D.R. Cox, and L. Billard. 1987. "Incubation Period of AIDS in Patient Infected via Blood Transfusion." *Nature* August 20–26:328(6132): 719–721.
Monmaney, T. 1988. "The AIDS Threat: Who's at Risk?" *Newsweek,* March 14, pp. 42–44.
Moss, R.J., and S.H. Miles. 1987. "AIDS and the Geriatrician." *Journal of the American Geriatrics Society* 35:460–464.
National Center for Health Statistics. 1987. "AIDS knowledge and attitudes for August, 1987. Provisional data from the National Health Interview Survey." *Advance Data From Vital and Health Statistics* No. 146.
Peterman, T.A., R.L. Stoneburner, J.R. Allen, H.W. Jaffe, and J.W. Curran. 1988. "Risk of Human Immunodeficiency Virus Transmission for Heterosexual Adults

with Transfusion-Associated Infections." *Journal of the American Medical Association* 258:55–58.
Pfeiffer, E., and G.C. Davis. 1972. "Determinants of Sexual Behavior in Middle and Old Age." *Journal of the American Geriatrics Society* 20:151–158.
Pfeiffer, E., A. Verwoerdt, and H.S. Wang. 1968. "Sexual Behavior in Aged Men and Women." *Archives of General Psychiatry* 19:753–758.
———. 1969. "The Natural History of Sexual Behavior in a Biologically Advantaged Group of Aged Individuals." *Journal of Gerontology* 24:193–198.
Pitchenik, A.E., M.A. Fischl, and T.J. Spira. 1983. "Acquired Immunodeficiency Syndrome in Low-Risk Patients: Evidence for Possible Transmission by an Asymptomatic Carrier." *Journal of the American Medical Association* 250:1310–1312.
Pitchenik, A.E., R.D. Shafron, R.M. Glasser, et al. 1984. "The Acquired Immunodeficiency Syndrome in the Life of a Hemophiliac." *Annals of Internal Medicine* 100:62–65.
Quinn, T.C., D. Glasser, R.O. Cannon, D.L. Matuszak, R.W. Dunning, R.L. Kline, C.H. Campbell, E. Israel, A.S. Fauci, and E.W. Hook. 1988. "Human Immunodeficiency Virus Infection Among Patients Attending Clinics for Sexually Transmitted Diseases." *New England Journal of Medicine* 318:197–203.
Schur, E.M. 1988. *The Americanization of Sex.* Philadelphia: Temple University Press.
Selwyn, P.A. 1986. *AIDS: What is Known.* New York: HP Publishing Company.
Singer, E., T.F. Rogers, and M. Corcoran. 1987. "The Polls—A Report: AIDS." *Public Opinion Quarterly* 51:580–595.
Stall, R., L. McKusick, J. Wiley, T.J. Coates, and D.G. Ostrow. 1986. "Alcohol and Drug Use During Sexual Activity and Compliance with Safe Sex Guidelines for AIDS: The AIDS Behavioral Research Project." *Health Education Quarterly* 13:359–371.
Starr, B.D. 1985. "Sexuality and Aging." Pp. 97–126 in C. Eisdorfer, M.P. Lawton, and G.L. Maddox (eds) *Annual Review of Gerontology and Geriatrics.* New York: Springer Publishing Company.
Starr, B.D., and M.B. Weiner. 1981. *The Starr-Weiner Report on Sex and Sexuality in the Mature Years.* New York: McGraw Hill.
Stehr-Green, J.K., R.C. Holman, J.M. Jason, and B.L. Evatt. 1988. "Hemophilia-Associated AIDS in the United States, 1981– September 1987." *American Journal of Public Health* 78:439–442.
Waksberg, J. 1978. "Sampling methods for random digit dialing." *Journal of the American Sociological Association* 77:40–46.
Weg, R.B. 1983. "Introduction: Beyond Intercourse and Orgasm." Pp. 1–37 in R.B. Weg (ed) *Sexuality in the Later Years.* New York: Academic Press.
Weinberg, M.S., and C. Williams. 1974. *Male Homosexuals.* New York: Oxford University Press.
Wish, E.D. February 1987. *Drug Use Forecasting: New York 1984 to 1986.* National Institute of Justice: Research in Action. Washington, D.C.

CHAPTER 4

The Social Epidemiology of AIDS and HIV Infection among Older Americans

Ron Stall, Joseph A. Catania, and Lance Pollack

This chapter is divided into three major sections that examine, from the perspective of social epidemiology, three selected aspects of the role played by older Americans in the AIDS epidemic. The first of these uses data on new AIDS cases reported to the Center for Disease Control (CDC) over a period of years, in order to investigate differences between younger and older people in sources of disease transmission; this section includes a crude demonstration of the persistence over the next decade of sizable numbers of AIDS cases among people over the age of 50. The second section reports findings from a study of gay and bisexual men in San Francisco, showing how the extent and sources of behavioral risk are changing for both older and younger men. The third section outlines a research design for use in constructing a model of care for older persons with AIDS. These three sections, though only loosely interrelated, together support the contention that AIDS is in part an age-defined disease, with older people constituting a substantial minority of the existing and probable future caseload.

Although one purpose of this chapter is to outline a few aspects of what is now known of the social epidemiology of AIDS among older Americans, the

Preparation of this chapter was supported in part by a contract from the National Institute on Aging, a National Institute of Mental Health grant (#MH 39353), and by a National Institute of Mental Health/National Institute on Drug Abuse Center Grant (#MH 42459).

This paper could not have been written without the participation of the men in the AIDS Behavioral Research Project and the participants in the Alternative Test Site study. The participants in these studies have patiently responded to questions regarding intimate life-style issues in the hope that the AIDS epidemic might be brought to an end. Drs. Susan Kegeles and Thomas J. Coates, of the Center for AIDS Prevention Studies, both provided valuable critiques of an earlier draft of this paper.

chapter also implicitly points to a larger research agenda for research on this topic. Identifying the transmission sources and the changes in these sources as they impinge on the elderly, and understanding how best to take care of older persons stricken with AIDS, are questions of central concern for the prevention and clinical care of AIDS among Americans in their middle and later years. Answers to such crucial research questions can only be hinted at in this brief chapter. Accordingly, the chapter has been written not only to outline some of the current findings on AIDS, but also to encourage other researchers to reexamine, refine, and specify these and other analyses, so that a continuing body of research can contribute to the larger public health research agenda (cf. Coates et al., 1987).

DISTRIBUTION OF NEW AIDS CASES IN THE U.S. BY AGE AND SOURCES OF TRANSMISSION

The tables in this section examine data for all new AIDS cases as reported annually to the Centers for Disease Control (CDC) since the start of the epidemic (pre-1982) through 1987. The tables exclude children under 13, and the data for 1987 are provisional as of January 4, 1988. As the data are presented, the focus is on older people's *share* of the new cases each year, on the *shares* of new cases attributed to the major sources of transmission, and on changes in these shares over time.

The word "share" is emphasized in order to call attention at the outset to the form of the analysis, and to the appropriate—as well as the inappropriate—interpretations of findings. The tables do *not* show incidence *rates* in the usual sense; that is, they do not show the proportions of those newly diagnosed with AIDS based on a denominator estimate of all gay/bisexual males, nor of all intravenous drug users, in a particular year. (Informative as such rates would be, reliable bases for these percentages are not available; e.g., we do not have at hand, by year and by age, the numbers of homosexual males, IV drug users, or transfusion recipients in the United States.) Instead, the tables presented here show *distributions of new AIDS cases*: that is, what the tables *do* show are the percentages who are IV drug users, for example, or who are age 50 and over, based on the newly diagnosed AIDS cases for each given year.

In addition to these analytical constraints, the CDC data themselves, although the best available, are subject to various well known limitations (e.g., incomplete reporting, the possibility of denial of membership in particular "risk categories," changing meanings of diagnostic terms as science has advanced), limitations which may be most pronounced in the pre-1982 data. Despite these interpretive cautions, the following descriptions of the several tables will illustrate the utility of examining distributions of new AIDS cases among age categories and among major sources of transmission, and they permit comparisons in these proportions from year to year. The analyses can be regarded as the beginning of a course set to uncover the changing associations between age and the course and sources of the AIDS epidemic.

Distribution of New Cases in the United States as a Whole

Table 4.1 describes the age distributions of all new adult/adolescent AIDS cases reported to the CDC each year up to January 4, 1988.

Notable in Table 4.1 are the changes over time in the total numbers of new cases (the bottom row of numbers in the table on which the percentages are based). There is an exponential rise in these numbers (an approximate redoubling) from the start of the epidemic through 1985. Although there may be a slowing in the subsequent rate of growth (the number for 1987 is provisional), the simple sum of the cases reported in this table (49,515) had already approached the number of American casualties during the Vietnam War, and will probably exceed that sad benchmark during 1988.

Within the body of the table, the age distributions of new AIDS cases have been remarkably consistent since the early days of the epidemic. In every year, nearly half of the new cases are concentrated in the age category 30 to 39. One-fifth are aged 13 to 29. Of special significance for this book, another one-fifth are aged 40 to 49 and, perhaps surprisingly, one-tenth are aged 50 and over. The remarkable stability of these distributions over time emphasizes the fact that age has clearly been an important predictor of AIDS diagnosis since the early days of the epidemic.

TABLE 4.1 New Cases of AIDS in U.S., Pre-1982 to 1987, Percent Distribution by Age

	Year of AIDS Diagnosis						
Age	Pre-1982 %	1982 %	1983 %	1984 %	1985 %	1986 %	1987 %
13–29	19.5	23.9	22.5	21.6	21.7	21.6	20.9
30–39	49.1	46.3	46.2	48.2	47.1	47.1	46.8
40–49	21.6	21.8	21.4	20.8	20.9	20.8	21.7
50+	9.9	8.1	9.9	9.4	10.3	10.6	10.5
Total cases = 100%	334	992	2754	5610	9956	14888	14981

Source: Centers for Disease Control (CDC) Surveillance Data as of January 4, 1988.

A reminder of the distributional form of this (and subsequent) tables is in order here as a cautionary note. It is important to keep in mind that this stability over time in the percentage distributions by age definitely does *not* mean that the *numbers* of cases in each category have not risen; rather, it means that no one age category has been increasing any more or less rapidly than the other age categories.

Table 4.2, which disregards age for the moment, shows how the new cases each year are distributed by the major sources of transmission. For every one of the years reported, key findings are persistent. Most notable is the marked predominance of cases attributed to the gay and bisexual male population, with intravenous (IV) drug users also constituting a substantial source. These two transmission categories have been of special concern during the early years of the epidemic. By contrast, hemophiliacs account for only 1.1% or less of the cases each year. Heterosexual transmission and blood transfusion are still relatively minor sources, but their future course is important to observe, as these sources may reach more generally into the population as a whole.

Over time, a few changes have appeared. The predominance of gay and bisexual males (including IV drug users) as a transmission source was most pronounced in the years before 1982, and somewhat less pronounced thereafter. There was little consistent change (save for pre-1982) in the relative importance of IV drug users. There are noticeable decreases up to 1984 in proportions of cases attributable to heterosexual transmission (though there may have been some misreporting early in the epidemic). By contrast, there has been a consistent increase in the proportions (though small) attributed to blood transfusions. (But again the caution: for all sources, even when the

TABLE 4.2 New Cases of AIDS in U.S., Pre-1982 to 1987, Percent Distribution by Major Sources of Transmission*

	Year of AIDS Diagnosis						
Transmission Category	Pre-1982 %	1982 %	1983 %	1984 %	1985 %	1986 %	1987 %
Gay/bisexual male	72.1	64.9	64.2	67.2	68.3	67.8	65.7
IV drug user	12.5	17.3	18.9	17.3	17.5	16.7	19.0
Gay/bisexual IV drug user	6.9	9.6	10.2	9.2	7.3	7.8	6.9
Hemophiliac	.6	.6	.5	1.0	1.1	1.1	1.1
Heterosexual	7.5	6.8	4.8	3.7	3.6	4.0	4.4
Transfusion	.3	.8	1.5	1.6	2.3	2.5	2.9
Total cases = 100%	319	960	2679	5474	9730	14478	14360

* Cases attributed to "other" categories of transmission (1515 cases, or 3.1% of the 48,000 cases reported) are omitted from Tables 4.2 through 4.4.

Source: Centers for Disease Control (CDC) Surveillance Data as of January 4, 1988.

percentages show a relative "decrease," the absolute numbers have tended to increase steadily.)

Distribution of New Cases within Age Categories

Tables 4.1 and 4.2 report data separately for age and for transmission category and can thus obscure important age-specific patterns. Yet it is interesting to learn, for example, what patterns characterize those in the middle and later years. To explore such questions, Tables 4.3 and 4.4 show breakdowns by age of the data on transmission categories from Table 4.2.

Table 4.3 shows, for a single year only, 1987, age differences in the distributions of these categories. (These data will appear again in Table 4.4, but it is instructive to examine age differences separately for the most recent year first.) Among the newly diagnosed cases in every age category, gay and bisexual males constitute the predominant transmission category; this predominance is most pronounced among those aged 40 to 49 (71.9%). IV drug use is relatively highest among those aged 30 to 39 (23.2%), but it is notably low (8.3%) among the new cases at the oldest ages (50+), where it is outdistanced by the 17.3% attributed to blood transfusion.

Table 4.4 carries the analysis one step further in order to observe the time trends behind these age differences in distribution of transmission categories. Table 4.4 shows the distribution for each year of the epidemic within each of the four age strata (in panels A, B, C, and D, respectively). That AIDS is a disease governed to no small degree by age-related phenomena is clearly apparent in the age-related differences in sources of transmission.

TABLE 4.3 New Cases of AIDS in U.S. by Age, 1987 Only, Percent Distribution by Major Source of Transmission

	Age			
Transmission Category	20–29* %	30–39 %	40–49 %	50+ %
Gay/bisexual male	65.4	63.2	71.9	65.8
IV drug user	16.6	23.2	17.3	8.3
Gay/bisexual IV drug user	8.8	8.2	4.7	1.9
Hemophiliac	1.4	.5	.9	2.0
Heterosexual	6.8	4.0	3.0	4.6
Transfusion	1.1	.9	2.2	17.3
Total Cases = 100%	2947	6787	3124	1450

* Tables 4.3 and 4.4 exclude the small number aged 13–19.

Source: Centers for Disease Control (CDC) Surveillance Data as of January 4, 1988.

TABLE 4.4 New Cases of AIDS in U.S., Pre-1982 to 1987, Percent Distributions within Age Categories

	Year of AIDS Diagnosis						
Transmission Category	Pre-1982 %	1982 %	1983 %	1984 %	1985 %	1986 %	1987 %
A. For Ages 20–29							
Gay/bisexual male	53.2	49.8	57.4	61.7	64.9	67.0	65.4
IV drug user	16.1	21.3	20.1	16.7	17.5	14.2	16.6
Gay/bisexual IV drug user	11.3	12.2	11.7	12.4	9.7	10.1	8.8
Hemophiliac	1.6	.5	.3	1.0	1.1	1.4	1.4
Heterosexual	17.7	15.8	10.0	7.5	5.7	6.5	6.8
Transfusion	0.0	.5	.5	.7	1.0	.9	1.1
Total cases = 100%	62	221	598	1155	2058	3081	2947
B. For Ages 30–39							
Gay/bisexual male	71.7	64.8	61.6	65.1	65.7	65.2	63.2
IV drug user	16.4	20.3	21.9	21.2	21.3	20.8	23.2
Gay/bisexual IV drug user	6.3	10.2	12.0	10.0	8.2	9.1	8.2
Hemophiliac	0.0	0.0	.2	.6	.7	.5	.5
Heterosexual	5.7	4.7	3.7	2.9	3.6	3.7	4.0
Transfusion	0.0	0.0	.5	.3	.5	.6	.9
Total cases = 100%	159	449	1249	2651	4634	6873	6787
C. For Ages 40–49							
Gay/bisexual male	82.4	76.0	73.6	75.7	77.1	75.6	71.9
IV drug user	5.9	11.1	15.1	13.6	13.7	14.5	17.3
Gay/bisexual IV drug user	4.4	8.7	7.6	6.9	5.2	5.2	4.7
Hemophiliac	0.0	.5	.5	1.0	.9	.7	.9
Heterosexual	5.9	2.9	2.5	2.4	2.0	2.4	3.0
Transfusion	1.5	1.0	.7	.5	1.0	1.6	2.2
Total cases = 100%	68	208	568	1134	2023	3005	3124
D. For Ages 50+							
Gay/bisexual male	89.7	81.6	73.4	73.0	70.6	66.8	65.8
IV drug user	0.0	5.3	9.0	7.3	7.8	8.0	8.3
Gay/bisexual IV drug user	6.9	1.3	3.9	2.8	1.9	2.6	1.9
Hemophiliac	3.4	5.3	1.2	2.0	2.4	2.1	2.0
Heterosexual	0.0	1.3	2.7	2.6	1.9	3.6	4.6
Transfusion	0.0	5.3	9.8	12.3	15.4	17.0	17.3
Total cases = 100%	29	76	256	504	975	1462	1450

Source: Centers for Disease Control (CDC) Surveillance Data as of January 4, 1988.

- As shown in Table 4.4 among those younger than 30 with AIDS, the proportion of gay/bisexual male cases has tended to climb. However, for every other age category, the proportion of cases attributable to male homosexual transmission has shown a distinct tendency to decline.
- The proportion of cases attributable to intravenous drug use has tended to rise among those in their thirties and forties. Among those aged 50 or older,

the proportion of such cases, which is lower than at any other stage of life, has remained fairly stable in recent years.

- Transfusion cases are rare among people with AIDS younger than 50, but have increased steadily and markedly among those older than 50.
- Those aged 50 or older are the only age category in which the proportion of AIDS cases attributable to heterosexual transmission has tended to increase.

These unique characteristics of the epidemic among different age categories suggest that prevention efforts and models of care may have to be specialized in order for such programs to be effective. For persons older than 50, potentially useful clues derive from the findings that proportions of cases drawn from among gay/bisexual men have been decreasing, whereas proportions attributable to blood transfusions and heterosexual contact have been increasing. At the same time, future programs must be guided by the finding that new cohorts of AIDS victims are being added to the burden of care at every age, and that at every age the numbers of new persons with AIDS (PWA) are increasing year by year. Moreover, given the incubation period that precedes the full-blown disease, it is obvious that prevention efforts must be made at every age to forestall the spread of HIV infection.

Persistence of AIDS among Older People of the Future

Predicting the future incidence of AIDS is surprisingly difficult (see Hyman & Stanley, forthcoming), and such attempts occasionally yield confidence intervals with an infinite upper boundary (Kalbfleisch, 1988). Predictions of the future AIDS caseload must at a minimum be based on accurate measures of the incubation period of the disease, the number of infected persons within a population, and the time of infection for antibody-positive persons. These measures are required even if we are to predict onset of disease among those already infected, without regard to future HIV infection. Although some crude estimates for each of these variables have been made, it cannot be said that any one of these estimates has been firmly established. Nor have any specialized estimates of these variables been agreed upon for specific age levels, and the opportunity to gather some critical data necessary for incidence estimates (e.g., time of onset of HIV infection) may have been lost for most populations. For these and other reasons, only very crude estimates of the future AIDS caseload among those aged 50 or greater can be attempted (see the chapter in this volume by Manton and Singer).

Although there are formidable difficulties in estimating the future burden of AIDS among the elderly, such estimates are of enormous value in health care planning. For this reason, an estimate of AIDS incidence over the next decade will be calculated, although this will admittedly be a very crude estimate. We hope that this preliminary attempt will inspire further work in modeling the future incidence of AIDS within older populations.

This exercise began with the working estimate that some 1 to 1.5 million Americans of all ages—call it 1.25 million—are infected with the HIV virus; this estimate was provided at the Public Health Service Conference at Coolfont, West Virginia (reviewed in DHHS, 1987). At the time, this estimate was consistent with projections from the contemporary AIDS caseload and was recommended as a reasonable basis for health planning purposes (DHHS, 1987; Institute of Medicine, 1986).

The next step was to estimate the number of Americans with HIV infection who were over the age of 50. Under the untested assumption that the proportion of older Americans infected with HIV in a given year is the same as the proportion actually diagnosed in that year as having AIDS (i.e., 10% as in Table 4.1 above), we then set the number as roughly 125,000 Americans over the age of 50 with HIV infection. (We have no basis for judging whether this is an overestimate or an underestimate.)

Further assumptions were that, in the absence of other information, all of these current infections occurred within the previous month; and that, contrary to reality, no further infections would occur among those nearing or past age 50. Another assumption was that a cure for AIDS will not be found over the next decade.

The remaining questions were: How many of these HIV seropositives would develop AIDS, and how long would the incubation period be? As illustrative answers to these questions, we used estimates based on the observed outcomes of long-term HIV infection in a sample of gay men in the San Francisco City Clinic (Hessol et al., 1988). In the early days of the epidemic, it had been hoped that only a small proportion of those infected with the virus would develop AIDS. Findings from this cohort now indicate, however, that 15% develop AIDS after 5 years of infection, 22% after 6 years, 34% after 7 years, 38% after 8 years, and 42% after 9 years of HIV infection. Moreover, among the gay men in this cohort infected with HIV for an average of 9 years, in addition to the 42% diagnosed with AIDS, another 47% have been diagnosed with associated opportunistic infections (symptoms earlier described as indicative of "ARC": oral candidiasis, hairy leukoplakia or generalized lymphadenopathy). Thus only 11% of the original cohort had no AIDS-related symptoms at all after 9 years of infection. Although it is believed that even this small proportion of the cohort will continue to dwindle over time, for present purposes we assume that no further AIDS-related symptoms will appear during the 10th year, and that the time period for development of the disease is the same for those over 50 as for the younger gay men in the San Francisco sample. Since further progression of the disease is almost certain to occur in this sample over the remaining year of the next decade, and since the incubation period may well be shorter among older than younger persons, these assumptions are likely to underestimate the future caseload of AIDS among the elderly.

Given these assumptions and estimates, then, we proceed to calculate the likely number of AIDS cases resulting over the next 10 years from the 125,000 Americans over the age of 50 who were HIV-seropositive in 1986. Using the San Francisco City Clinic data as a guide, we can conservatively estimate that 42% (or 52,500) of these HIV seropositives will be diagnosed with AIDS over the coming decade, while another 47% (or 58,750) will be diagnosed with associated opportunistic infections. Only 11% (or 13,750) of the original cohort can be expected to remain asymptomatic during this time period. In other words, at the very minimum, we estimate that over the next decade the cumulative number of new cases of AIDS over the age of 50 will exceed the total number (49,515, see Table 4.1) of adult Americans of all ages already diagnosed with AIDS from the beginning of the epidemic until 1988.

What is most sobering about this conclusion is that every effort has been made to generate a conservative estimate. That is, the assumptions—that no further HIV transmission is occurring, that the proportion of AIDS diagnoses does not increase in the 10th year after infection, that the incubation period for the onset of AIDS among older people is the same as for younger people, and that all infection has occurred within the recent past—are all likely to underestimate the coming burden of AIDS cases among those over the age of 50.

Both the unique epidemiological profile of AIDS among older people and the large number of older Americans who will undoubtedly develop the disease in the future ensure that AIDS will become a topic of increasing concern to those interested in the health and care of older Americans.

SEXUAL RISK FOR HIV INFECTION AMONG GAY MEN IN SAN FRANCISCO

The CDC data for 1987 presented in the foregoing section (Table 4.3 above) have identified two major risk categories for people over age 50: gay and bisexual men (accounting for 65.8% of new cases) and transfusion-related cases (accounting for another 17.3% of new cases). Together these two risk categories account for some 83% of the AIDS diagnoses among people over 50. Since the advent of HIV antibody testing of donated blood, the risk of further AIDS infection attributable to transfusions has become markedly reduced. Thus, two assumptions can be made concerning the prevention of HIV infection among older Americans: (1) that it is among older transfusion recipients and gay men that prevention efforts should be initially concentrated, and (2) that sexual behaviors will be the means whereby further HIV transmission from infected persons within these transmission categories is most likely to spread. This section describes how the extent of risk for HIV infection and changes in this risk differ by age among gay men in San Francisco. (See the chapter by Catania et al. for a parallel description of sexual risk for HIV infection among older transfusion recipients in the Bay Area.)

Data presented here are drawn from a single study, the "AIDS Behavioral Research Project," as described, for example, in McKusick, Hortsman, and Coates (1985) and McKusick et al. (1985). This research project was originally designed to determine how the AIDS epidemic was influencing gay men's psychological adjustment and sexual behavior. A survey questionnaire has been administered to this cohort semiannually since November 1983 until November 1985, and annually thereafter, thus providing one of the longest continuing studies of risk measurement of any of the behavioral HIV studies of gay/bisexual men.

The Sample

Men were recruited opportunistically from four sources: (1) bathhouses, (2) gay bars, (3) advertisements requesting participation from gay men who found their sexual partners from neither bathhouses nor bars, and (4) lists of gay male couples who had participated in other research projects.

Though not representational, these opportunistic samples from relatively distinct subgroups of gay men were designed to give a picture of the varied types of changes in sexual behavior that gay men have made in response to the AIDS epidemic in San Francisco. Initially, this method of recruitment resulted in a sample with higher overall numbers of sexual partners than were found at about the same time in two other probability samples of gay men in San Francisco (Anderson & Levy, 1985; Research Decisions Corporation, 1984). However, by May 1985 the behavior reported in the opportunistic sample closely approximated that reported in a random telephone survey of gay and bisexual men in San Francisco at about the same time (Research Decisions Corporation, 1985). Thus, the data presented here give useful indications of behavioral adaptations that have occurred within the gay male community of San Francisco.

Scale of Behavioral Risk among Gays

At each interview a detailed measure of participation during the past 30 days in a wide variety of sexual behaviors was constructed. From these ongoing measures we have used, with minor modifications, a scale developed by the Chicago Multi-Center AIDS Cohort Study Group (Joseph et al., 1987) for predicting HIV seroconversion over time among gay/bisexual men. This scale has four categories. Those at "no risk" were celibate. Those at "low risk" had anal sex with a condom within the bounds of a monogamous relationship or, if not monogamous, no anal sex at all. Those in the "modified high risk" category had anal sex without a condom within the bounds of a monogamous relationship and, if not monogamous, had anal sex only while using a condom. Those at "high risk" had anal sex without a condom and outside of monogamous relationships. This scale has been modified to include insertive, as well as receptive, anal sex for all forms of anal sex without use of a condom.

Scale of Behavioral Risk

Table 4.5 shows how gay/bisexual men within each of four age categories in the sample were distributed along the scale of behavioral risk at three survey waves: 1984, 1985, and 1986. (Age categories have been constructed so that individuals can change categories as they grow older from one wave to another.)

The trend over the 2-year period shows pronounced decreases in the proportions with high-risk behavior. Regardless of age, these men were about twice as likely to be at high risk in 1984 as they were 2 years later. Behavioral

TABLE 4.5 Trends in Sexual Risk for HIV Infection among Gay and Bisexual Men in San Francisco from 1984 to 1986 (Row percentages)

Age	Numbers in parentheses = 100%	Risk category			
		No	Low	Mod High	High
19–29					
1984	(173)	11.6	24.3	17.9	46.2
1985	(115)	10.4	34.8	28.7	26.1
1986	(65)	7.7	38.5	35.4	18.5
30–39					
1984	(340)	10.6	29.1	17.4	42.9
1985	(320)	15.6	36.3	22.8	25.3
1986	(294)	16.7	37.8	24.5	21.1
40–49					
1984	(146)	13.7	39.0	11.6	35.6
1985	(151)	20.5	41.1	18.5	19.9
1986	(146)	17.1	44.5	23.3	15.1
50+					
1984	(45)	24.4	26.7	17.8	31.1
1985	(47)	29.8	34.0	21.3	14.9
1986	(44)	18.2	40.9	25.0	15.9

Source: The AIDS Behavior Risk Project.

risk reductions of this magnitude over so brief a time period are probably unique in the public health prevention literature.

Moreover, there is clearly a relationship between age and risk (although the numbers used as bases for the percentages are small in the oldest age category). This relationship between the four levels of risk and the four age categories was most pronounced in 1984, prior to the overall trend toward less risky behavior. For these 3 years at least, these data point to a weakening over time of the relationship between age and risk (chi square in 1984 $p < .03$; in 1985 $p < .07$; and in 1986 $p < .41$). Even at the oldest ages (50+), though the proportion at high risk in 1984 was clearly lower than at younger ages, by 1986 this age discrepancy had become reduced.

Number of Contacts

This scale of risk behavior, as presented in Table 4.5, is essentially quantitative: it does not take into account numbers of partners or frequency of contact. Accordingly, we have supplemented the analysis by using a simple summary measure of the number of times each respondent had unprotected anal intercourse with a nonmonogamous partner. The age categories from Table 4.5 were dichotomized into men younger than 39 and those 40 and older.

This analysis shows that at each wave of data collection the younger gay men had higher mean numbers of high risk sexual encounters than did the older men and all these age differences were statistically significant at the .02 level or better, using a *t*-test. In November 1984 the younger gay men had a mean of 2.4 unprotected contacts, while the older men had a mean of 1.4 such contacts. At Wave 2 (in November 1985) the mean number of high-risk contacts for the younger group had been reduced to 1.1, and for the older men to 0.6. By November 1986 the younger men had a mean of 0.9 high-risk contacts, while the older men had a mean of only 0.4. Thus at each wave of data collection the younger men had approximately twice the mean number of high risk sexual contacts as did those 40 and over.

Moreover, over the 2-year period men in both age categories showed a strong trend toward reducing the numbers of high-risk sexual contacts. This finding, though taken from a single localized sample, constitutes further evidence of sharp changes in the behavior of gay and bisexual males.

It should also be pointed out that the self-reported behavioral data from the AIDS Behavioral Research Project replicated the impression gained from CDC data described above. That is, the behavioral data indicate that gay men younger than 29 were slower than the older men to reduce their participation in high-risk behaviors. As late as 1984, nearly one-half of the younger gay men could still be classified as high risk (Table 4.5). Similarly, the CDC data indicate that the proportion of new AIDS cases attributable to gay/bisexual contacts has been uniquely increasing among the youngest age group, also supporting the contention that risk reduction among younger gay men has been slower than among older gay men. There is cause for policy concern here, especially since the long incubation period before onset of the AIDS disease means that many of those diagnosed with AIDS during their twenties had already become infected with the virus as teenagers.

Designs for behavioral risk reduction among gay men of all ages have been described (see, e.g., Stall, Coates, & Hoff, 1988). In addition, it should be noted that the behavioral data cited here tell nothing of the levels of sexual risk in areas outside of the major urban "gay ghettos." Further age-specific analyses, utilizing data from gay men who live outside of the major coastal gay communities, are needed to determine whether the impressions gained from the gay community of San Francisco also hold for other parts of the nation. It goes without saying that these same types of research should also be attempted among the American heterosexual population.

DEVELOPING A MODEL OF CARE FOR OLDER PERSONS WITH AIDS

As the third aspect of the AIDS epidemic to be considered, we turn to the needs for care among older persons with AIDS, a topic to which little attention has yet been devoted. This section outlines a design for research that could be useful in developing a model of care for elderly persons with AIDS (see also the chapter in this book by Crystal).

Our primary objective in developing such a model is to investigate the experiences of older persons with AIDS in finding out about sources of care, their experience in getting care, the amount of care that they receive, their perceptions of that care, and what care they are not getting but still need. "Care" will be defined in a way that is broader than the care received through the medical care system: It will also include care received through public agencies and through kin and social networks, as well as self-care. Strategies can also be devised to estimate, through this study, the cost of care for different types of AIDS patients, with measures of cost-effectiveness of care incorporating patient perceptions of the value of that care.

To meet this objective, the research design we propose is a modification of a standard case-control epidemiological study to include both quantitative and qualitative data regarding the search for care for different types of older patients. The quantitative data will be used to identify any differences in the search for care between different types of patients; the qualitative data will then be used to investigate why such differences exist. The two types to be compared will be those most prevalent among older persons with AIDS: gay men and transfusion cases. The controls will be drawn from a diagnostic category similar to AIDS in allowing a sizable survival time after diagnosis and in requiring intensive and largely low-technology care. To meet these criteria, we have selected cancer patients. Controls will also be drawn so that they are comparable in respect to socioeconomic status, ethnicity, sex, and age.

The analysis of data will be so constructed that the experiences of each type of AIDS patient in obtaining care can be compared to their respective controls. In this manner we can learn about older people, first, what is different about having AIDS rather than another life-threatening illness. Secondly, we can learn what is different about having AIDS as a result of a stigmatizing behavior (i.e., gay/bisexual contact) from a nonstigmatizing experience (i.e., a blood transfusion). Here the two types of AIDS patients can be compared with each other and also with the cancer controls. Findings should be particularly valuable in identifying the unique needs of nonstigmatized elderly patients that are above and beyond those met by the relatively well-defined model of care now available for gay men.

It is our hope that, by such comparison of the care experiences and costs of older AIDS patients with those of similar patients with another life-threatening illness, we shall be in a better position to construct a cost-effective and humane model of care to meet the needs of older persons with AIDS.

DISCUSSION

AIDS has been defined by age since the early days of the epidemic. The disease has primarily manifested among those younger than 40, although a stable proportion of persons with AIDS is drawn from those over the age of 50. Further, it may be that the types of behavioral risks for HIV infection are changing at proportionately different rates over time among persons in different age categories. The extent of sexual risk among gay men is strongly predicted by age, younger men in San Francisco having been at greatest behavioral risk of HIV transmission until rather recently. The frequency of sexual risk among heterosexuals is also believed to be associated with chronological age (Gagnon, 1989).

It should also be pointed out that the self-reported behavioral data from the AIDS Behavioral Research Project replicate the findings implicit in the Centers for Disease Control Surveillance Data. The behavioral data indicate that gay men younger than 29 were the slowest to reduce their participation in high risk behaviors. As late as 1984, nearly one-half of the youngest gay men could be classified as high risk on the basis of their sexual behaviors during the previous month alone. The Centers for Disease Control Surveillance Data indicate that the proportion of the AIDS caseload attributable to homosexual contact is uniquely tending to increase among the youngest age group, also supporting the contention that risk reduction among younger gay men has been slower than among older gay men. Since the incubation period for the onset of full-blown AIDS is so long, it is possible that many of those diagnosed with AIDS in their twenties were infected with HIV as teenagers. Designing effective HIV prevention campaigns for gay male teenagers and young adults should be an urgent priority. To restrict such campaigns (e.g., through Congressional action) without an evaluation of these approaches in a sense requires public health practitioners to passively measure the phenomena of young men becoming infected with a deadly virus while denying public health workers effective means to prevent continuing tragedy.

Both AIDS surveillance and behavioral data are useful in the identification of subcategories at particularly high risk of new HIV infection. The identification of such categories can be useful in the design of specialized prevention campaigns. As previously indicated, one of these categories is young gay men. AIDS surveillance and alternative test site behavior risk data both suggest that the sexual partners of older transfusion recipients are also at high risk of HIV exposure. Consequently the content of prevention messages should be appropriate to the age levels of the target population. For example, health education messages regarding the dangers of high-risk sexual behavior with multiple sex partners may be less appropriate for target populations of older persons than are messages regarding the potential dangers of unprotected sex with persons who have had a blood transfusion prior to 1985.

In part, the relationship between age and the AIDS epidemic has to do with the importance of age predicting the kinds of risk behaviors in which individuals are likely to engage. Specifically, young people are more likely to explore nontraditional ways to have sex or use drugs than are older people, while the elderly are more likely to have had blood transfusions previous to 1985 or to have unprotected sex with someone who has. Similarly, if the experiences of gay men in San Francisco are generalizable to other populations, the young are more likely to engage in increased amounts of sexual behaviors involving risk for HIV infection. If these contentions are supported by further analyses, then the relationship between age and risk for HIV infection can be used to define both the populations in need of specialized HIV prevention efforts and the content of the prevention strategies.

Two metaphors are commonly used to describe the AIDS epidemic. One of these is the iceberg, the other a mosaic. Both are also applicable to the study of AIDS among older Americans. Regarding the first metaphor—that of the iceberg—it is commonly pointed out that the current caseload is only a small fraction of the cases to be expected in the future, even if no further HIV transmission occurs. This is also, tragically, the case among older Americans as well. The second metaphor—that of the mosaic—is used to describe the unique characteristics of the epidemic as it becomes manifest within different populations. The use of this metaphor is meant to convey the idea that the AIDS epidemic is not uniform across different populations and is perhaps more accurately conceived as a conglomeration of smaller epidemics, each with its own specific mode of transmission resulting from the patterning of risk behaviors within very different populations. Thus the epidemic among gay men in San Francisco is very different from that among sub-Saharan Africans, and both of these subepidemics appear to be different from that found among urban intravenous drug users. Both the CDC AIDS surveillance data and the San Francisco studies of behavioral risk suggest that older Americans are another tile in the growing mosaic that is the AIDS epidemic.

REFERENCES

Anderson, R.D., and J. Levy. 1985. "Prevalence of Antibodies to AIDS-Associated Retrovirus in Single Men in San Francisco." *Lancet* 8422:217.

Coates, T.J., R. Stall, J.S. Mandel, A. Boccellari, J.L. Sorensen, E.F. Morales, S.F. Morin, J. Wiley, and L. McKusick. 1987. "AIDS: A Psychosocial Research Agenda." *Annals of Behavioral Medicine* 9:21–28.

Department of Health and Human Services (DHHS). 1987. *A Review of Current Knowledge and Plans for Expansion of HIV Surveillance Activities: A Report to the Domestic Policy Council.* Department of Health and Human Services, Public Health Service, Centers for Disease Control, Washington, D.C., November 30, 1987.

Gagnon, John H. 1989. "Sexuality Across the Life Course in the United States." Pp. 500–536 in C.F. Turner, H.G. Miller, and L.E. Moses (eds.) *AIDS Sexual Behavior and Intravenous Drug Use.* Washington, DC: National Academy Press.

Hessol, N., G. Rutherford, P. O'Malley, L. Doll, W. Darrow, and H. Jaffe. 1988. *The Natural History of Human Immunodeficiency Virus Infection in a Cohort of Homosexual and Bisexual Men: A 7-Year Prospective Study.* Paper presented at the IV International AIDS Conference, Stockholm, Sweden, June, 1988.

Hyman, J.M., and E.A. Stanley. Forthcoming. "Using mathematical models to understand the AIDS epidemic." *Mathematical Biosciences.*

Institute of Medicine, National Academy of Sciences. 1986. *Confronting AIDS: Directions for Public Health, Health Care, and Research.* Washington, D.C.: National Academy Press.

Joseph, J., S. Montgomery , R. Kessler, D. Ostrow, D. Emmons, and J. Phair. 1987. *Two-Year Longitudinal Study of Behavioral Risk Reduction in a Cohort of Homosexual Men.* Paper presented at the III International AIDS Conference, Washington, D.C., June, 1987.

Kalbfleisch, J. 1988. "Discussion of Medley, Anderson, Cox and Billard in *Nature.*" Paper presented at the biweekly epidemiology seminar at the Center for AIDS Prevention Studies, San Francisco.

McKusick, L., W. Horstman, and T.J. Coates. 1985. "AIDS and Sexual Behavior Reported by Gay Men in San Francisco." *American Journal of Public Health,* 75:493–496.

McKusick, L., J. Wiley, T. Coates, R. Stall, G. Saika, S. Morin, K. Charles, W. Hortsman, and M. Conant. 1985. "Reported Changes, in the Sexual Behavior of Men at Risk for AIDS, San Francisco, 1982–1984—The AIDS Behavioral Research Project." *Public Health Reports* 100:622–625.

Research Decisions Corporation. 1984. *Designing an Effective AIDS Prevention Campaign Strategy for San Francisco: Results from the First Probability Sample of an Urban Gay Male Community.* Report prepared for the San Francisco AIDS Foundation, San Francisco.

Stall, R., T. Coates, and C. Hoff. 1988. "Behavioral Risk Reduction for HIV Infection Among Gay and Bisexual Men: A Review of the Results from the United States." *American Psychologist* 43(11):878–885.

CHAPTER 5

HIV Transmission Risks of Older Heterosexuals and Gays

Joseph A. Catania, Heather Turner,
Susan M. Kegeles, Ron Stall, Lance Pollack,
Sherry E. Spitzer, and Thomas J. Coates

Preventing transmission of human immunodeficiency virus (HIV) is the single most important AIDS-related public health goal. In pursuing this goal, investigators have focused on those age groups representing the majority of AIDS cases during the early years of the epidemic in the United States: adolescents and those in early adulthood (see the chapter in this volume by Stall, Catania, & Pollack). However, AIDS represents a global health problem that confronts people of all races and sexual orientations and all ages. In line with the theme of this book, greater attention should be paid to the HIV transmission risks and prevention needs of late-middle-aged and elderly individuals, which will predictably increase with further spread of the epidemic.

This chapter deals with primary prevention of HIV infection, with special reference to the older population. It begins by drawing attention to two comparatively neglected sources of transmission of the virus: blood transfusions and heterosexual relationships. Both of these sources are important at the later ages. Older individuals (aged 50+) have exhibited a significant increase in transfusion-related cases from 1982 to 1987 (Peterman, Jaffe, Feorino, et al., 1985; see also the chapter by Stall, Catania, & Pollack in this volume). As of 1987, transfusion-related cases stood as the second largest risk group among older people. Similarly, older individuals have shown a steadily increasing trend over time in prevalence of AIDS cases attributable to heterosexual transmission. Because of the long lag time between HIV infection and

This research was supported in part by NIMH Grant No. MH39553 and NIMH/NIDA Center Grant No. MH42459.

onset of symptoms (Curran, Jaffe, Hardy, et al., 1988), these rates reflect infection patterns of 5 to 7 years ago. They do not reflect the current prevalence of infection.

Another specific focus of this chapter is on the processes through which sexual behaviors and attitudes can lead to infection. In order to provide a framework for primary prevention, existing psychosocial knowledge and theories about behavior change are formulated as a conceptual model of AIDS risk reduction. In the closing sections of the chapter, this model is used as a guide for specifying areas of needed research.

BLOOD TRANSFUSIONS AS A SOURCE OF INFECTION

Blood transfusions are, unfortunately, an extremely efficient method of transmitting HIV (Anderson et al., 1986; Berglund et al., 1988; Menitove, 1986; Ward et al., 1987). Moreover, a small number of seropositive donors may infect a relatively large number of recipients (see Anderson et al., 1986; Berglund et al., 1988). Not surprisingly, older people—with their vulnerability to chronic diseases and disabilities requiring transfusions—are reported to have been frequent recipients of infected blood (Berglund et al., 1988; Peterman et al., 1988).

Scope of the Problem

To gain an appreciation of the potential magnitude of the HIV-related blood transfusion problem among older people, we need estimates of the number of older individuals who may have received infected blood. However, accurate estimates are difficult to derive for many reasons, including the deaths of transfusion recipients prior to the availability of HIV testing, repeated transfusions of the same person over time, and the impossible task of ex post facto testing of blood supplies for the prescreening years prior to 1985 (National Academy of Sciences, 1986). Furthermore, geographic differences in the distribution of infected blood and in the characteristics of recipient populations increase the uncertainty of any estimates of the number of people, particularly older individuals, infected through transfusion. In addition, current estimates of the total number of HIV infections due to blood transfusions set upper limits that, for all practical purposes, are meaningless because they approach infinity (as shown by Kalbfleisch & Lawless, 1988; see also Peterman et al., 1987).

Although we cannot estimate reliably the number of older transfusers infected with HIV, we can gain some appreciation of the potential magnitude of the problem by estimating the number of older people who received blood transfusions during the critical period from 1978 to March 1985—the approximately 7 years that the U.S. blood supply was contaminated. Such an estimate would provide the theoretical upper limit of those older transfusers who could have been infected by HIV. Although admittedly crude, one estimate of the number of people aged 50 and older who received blood transfusions during this period can be based on Friedman, Burn, and Schork's (1980) national study of transfusion trends for a 6-month period in 1979. Extrapolating from Friedman et al.'s data (collected in 1979) yields a cumulative total, for the critical period, of 253,064 older people (aged 50 and over) receiving blood transfusions. This figure must be viewed with great caution since it does not take into account alterations in medical care practices, population changes, death of recipients, or rehospitalizations. Nevertheless it is sufficient to indicate that there may be a large population at risk. It is imperative that research be conducted to accurately estimate the number of older people who may be at risk from HIV-infected blood, most immediately for those older people living in geographic areas of high HIV infection (e.g., California, New York, Florida).

Transmission to Sexual Partners

Since 1985 HIV infection through blood transfusion in the United States has become a limited transmission route, given efforts to screen the blood supply. However, those people already infected by blood transfusion form a nucleus for additional HIV transmission, and several studies have documented instances of HIV transmission from seropositive transfusion recipients to their sexual partners (Anderson et al., 1986; Berglund et al., 1988; L'age-Stehr et al., 1985; Peterman et al., 1988). In one study, Peterman and colleagues (1988) found 8% of the older male (2/25; 95% confidence limits, 1% to 26%) and 18% of the older female (10/55; 95% confidence limits, 9% to 31%) sexual partners of seropositive blood recipients to be HIV-positive. In addition, in this sample seropositive wives were even older than seronegative wives (median ages, 62 and 54 years respectively), suggesting that wives of transfusion recipients may be more likely to become infected if they are closer to their sixties than their fifties.

Early findings from our own ongoing study of people seeking antibody testing have produced a startling picture of the sexual practices and knowledge of older transfusers. (This study, supported by the National Institute of Mental Health, is conducted by Coates, Kegeles, & Catania.) In this sample, among 57 older participants (50 to 78 years old) 40% sought testing because they feared HIV infection from prior blood transfusions. These older respondents represented half of all individuals seeking testing for the reason that they feared infection from a blood transfusion. Despite the small sample size, preliminary analyses of the older transfusers have produced striking and consistent results both in respect to sexual practices and knowledge.

Among those older transfusers who answered questions about condom use ($n = 10$), none were using condoms during intercourse with their primary or secondary partners over the 6-month period prior to seeking testing. Consistent with this observation, the study by Peterman and associates (1988) found that none of the older heterosexual transfusers with HIV-positive sexual partners (median age for men was 72 and for women 62) had been using condoms since receiving their blood transfusions. In our sample, we also found that over half of older transfusers did not know that latex condoms can prevent HIV transmission.

In respect to knowledge, we found that, relative to older individuals who sought testing because of sexual concerns, older transfusers were significantly less likely to believe they could infect a sexual partner with HIV. The data suggest that older transfusers are not aware of the implications of their sexual behavior for HIV transmission, nor of the need for protective measures. One explanation for this low level of awareness may be that older transfusers become cognizant of their risk only after receiving notification from a hospital or personal physician. Indeed, many older people in our study arrived for testing with letters and prescriptions for antibody testing from their physicians or hospitals. This suggests that, prior to being notified, these people may not have been aware of their risk for infection and, therefore, had not appropriately modified their sexual behavior.

In short, our findings and those of Peterman and associates suggest that some older transfusion-infected individuals are unintentionally transmitting HIV to their sexual partners. This situation could account for the observed increase in heterosexual AIDS cases among older individuals (see the chapter by Stall, Catania, & Pollack in this volume). Underlying this transfusion scenario may be a failure of public health and news media messages to penetrate all AIDS risk groups equally. Further, there may be a tendency by some to deny altogether that older individuals are sexually active (cf. White & Catania, 1982), and, as a result, older transfusers may not be adequately advised to take safe sex precautions.

HETEROSEXUAL TRANSMISSION

Review of the literature on heterosexual transmission of HIV (Piot, Kreiss, Ndinya-Achola et al., 1987) leads to the following observations: On a worldwide basis, heterosexual HIV transmission is probably more common than homosexual transmission. Although the relative number of heterosexual

AIDS cases in the United States has been low, these cases comprise the fastest-growing group with AIDS. HIV can be transmitted through penis-in-vagina intercourse, and transmission is bidirectional, as demonstrated in a prospective study of the spouses of AIDS patients, where 42% of the wives and 38% of the husbands became HIV-positive over time.

Coital Frequency among Older People

Clearly, heterosexual HIV transmission occurs. However, do older heterosexuals engage in sexual activity often enough for efficient sexual transmission of HIV to occur from infected to noninfected partners? Table 5.1 summarizes data from two classic studies of older heterosexuals conducted respectively by Pfeiffer, Verwoerdt, and Davis (1972) and Martin (1975). Both studies indicated that the vast majority of the older participants were sexually active (save for older women, many of whom are widows.) Median activity levels as low as 2 to 4 times per month, as reported in these studies, may be sufficient for transmission given the wide variability in the number of exposures

TABLE 5.1 Coital Activity of Older Adults: Results from the Duke and Baltimore Longitudinal Studies

Pfeiffer, Verwoerdt, and Davis, 1972[a]	Men		Women	
	50s	60s	50s	60s
Coitally active in past year	94%	78	73	32
Coital frequency:				
=/> 4/month	60	32	35	10
=/> 10/month	14	4	7	2
N =	102	116	115	99
Married	98%		71%	

Martin, 1975[b]	Age Groups		
	50s	60s	70s
Coitally active in past year	94%	79	62
Coital frequency past 5 years (median/month)	4	2	2
N =	163	113	94

[a] Sample composed of middle class whites.
[b] Sample composed of middle class white married men; N = 362 who were 50+years, and N = 207 who were 60+years.

required to transmit HIV. Some individuals become infected after a single exposure, whereas others remain uninfected after hundreds of contacts (Padian, Marquis, Francis, et al., 1987; Piot et al., 1987). In fact, Peterman et al. (1988) found that older partners of HIV-infected blood recipients in his sample (median age, 62) had a higher prevalence of infection, despite lower levels of coital contacts (2.9 contacts per month), than did younger partners (median age 54), who had 4.6 contacts per month. In short, despite declining coital frequencies with age (for reviews, see Berezin, 1976; Ludeman, 1981; White & Catania, 1982), there is reason to believe that older individuals have intercourse at levels adequate for efficient HIV transmission.

Age-Related Biological Factors in Vulnerability

Certain biological changes with aging that may increase the efficiency of HIV transmission among older individuals relate to decreased immune system function with age and postmenopausal vaginal changes. There is widespread documentation of changes in a person's immune system function over time. In particular, the primary antibody response appears to decline with age (Makinodan, 1977). Declining immune system function could explain why older individuals have a lower median HIV incubation time than younger adults—5.8 vs. 7.3 years respectively (Kalbfleisch & Lawless, 1988). In addition, Peterman et al. (1988) suggest that older sex partners of HIV-infected transfusers are more likely to seroconvert than their younger counterparts. These observations, in conjunction with evidence suggesting that greater HIV infectivity facilitates sexual transmission (for review see Piot et al., 1987), reinforce the hypothesis that older heterosexuals can efficiently transmit HIV through sexual contact.

Further support comes from the tendency of postmenopausal women to experience a thinning of the vaginal wall due to estrogen loss and, therefore, to exhibit vaginal mucosal disruption during coitus (Weg, 1978, 1983). Since genital lesions are suspected to be a contributor to HIV infection (see the review by Piot et al., 1987), tears in an older woman's vaginal wall could provide this facilitative function. Thus, some older women may be at greater risk for HIV infection than others because of having more sites for viral entry.

Moreover, other sexually transmitted diseases (STDs) may serve as "cofactors" of HIV transmission (Piot et al., 1987), although such cofactors remain to be fully examined with respect to AIDS and older individuals. Approximately 3% of older men in developed countries are estimated to be infected with gonorrhea, and a prevalence of 1.5% for latent syphilis has been reported (Felstein, 1983), figures that are low relative to other age categories. However, older individuals' discomfort with discussing sex with physicians (Gendel, personal communication; White & Catania, 1982) may reduce the levels of reporting or of seeking treatment for STDs. Studies are needed to address the STD cofactor issue for the older population.

Age-Related Behavioral Risk Factors

Just as biological changes with age may affect older people's vulnerability to HIV infection, there are undoubtedly age-related sexual behaviors and life-style factors that influence transmission of the disease. Here again there is little firm information, either about older people or the United States population as a whole. Most of the available data are either out-of-date or derived from non-random samples, and past research has failed to determine the proportion or demographic characteristics of older people at risk. Although this paucity of information has been discussed elsewhere in this volume (see especially the chapter by Levy and Albrecht), a few key points are worth reemphasizing here.

Factors that increase the risk of AIDS include a variety of unsafe sexual practices, including the failure to use condoms. There are no data, however, that detail the extent of anal sex, mutual masturbation, oral sex, or use of sex toys among older people.

Risk of the disease is also affected by the number and character of relationships with sex partners. Engaging in sex with multiple partners may increase the risk of HIV infection (Curran et al., 1988), but how common is multiple-partner sex among older heterosexuals? The possibility that it may be becoming more common than it used to be is suggested by two studies that compare earlier cohorts of older heterosexuals with more recent cohorts (Downey, 1980; Dressel & Avant, 1983). The earlier cohorts reported a comparatively greater tendency toward monogamous sexual relationships, with somewhat less diversity within these relationships, whereas the more recent cohorts exhibited a comparatively higher prevalence of extramarital sexual activity than did their earlier counterparts. How generalizable to all older heterosexuals these findings are, however, and to what extent they identify a continuing trend has not been established.

In contrast to multiple-partner sex, monogamy—to the extent that it is the norm among most older people—would tend to limit the spread of the AIDS epidemic. Yet even with complete monogamy, lack of safe sex practices by those infected from other sources could in principle double the number of AIDS cases. Moreover, there is considerable doubt as to whether monogamy is "complete" in American society. Indeed, scattered research (e.g., Schlesinger, 1983) and anecdotal reports (Evelyn Gendel, UCSF Human Sexuality Clinic, personal communication, June, 1988) report that some older individuals belong to "Golden Swinger" clubs, and that others employ prostitutes of both sexes. The spread of infection may be inhibited by the increase in older age, particularly among women, of widowhood. However, widowhood does not invariably lead to sexual abstinence (Ludeman, 1981; White & Catania, 1982).

For the future, these and related clues must be intensively studied if we are to gain an understanding of HIV transmission in the heterosexual population. We also need to understand the sources of HIV transmission that predominate among older gay males (see Stall, Catania, & Pollack in this volume.)

OLDER GAY MEN AS A SOURCE OF TRANSMISSION

Since the start of the AIDS epidemic in the United States, gay and bisexual men have comprised the largest group of new AIDS cases each year, contributing 65% of the cases among older individuals in the CDC data for 1987. Sexual transmission of HIV has been the primary route of HIV infection for older gay and bisexual men. There is overwhelming evidence that gay men who practice unprotected anal sexual activity are at risk for transmitting HIV (Curran et al., 1988; Lifson, 1988). However, compared to their heterosexual counterparts, older gay men may be more knowledgeable about AIDS. For example, in our ongoing longitudinal study of older gay men over 90% knew that condoms prevent HIV transmission (unpublished results), whereas only half of older heterosexuals in our testing center study knew this fact. Older gay men have also, at least in San Francisco, reduced high-risk sexual behavior from 1984 to 1986.

Are the observed changes in high-risk sexual practices of older gay men from San Francisco generalizable? The gay community in San Francisco is often characterized as more cohesive and organized than gay communities in other parts of the country. This cohesiveness may be particularly salient for some older gay men who need a strong community base before "coming out" (Kelly, 1977; Kimmel, 1980), but it is possible that closeted older gay men are less influenced by changing sexual norms in the gay community and, therefore, continue to practice high-risk behaviors. Regional differences in the patterns and changes in sexual activities and attitudes of older gay and bisexual men are worthy of much further study.

Although most older gays have tended to reduce their high-risk behavior, a sizable minority continues to engage in unprotected anal intercourse. Even though these individuals may be engaging in high-risk activities within monogamous relationships and at lower frequencies than younger gays, these factors do not necessarily confer safety. An older gay couple who have been monogamous for 20 years may still be at risk when performing unprotected anal intercourse if one or both received blood transfusions between 1978 and 1985 or used infected IV needles. Moreover, as noted previously, low frequencies of sexual behavior do not necessarily protect this older population against sexual transmission of HIV.

Older gay or bisexual men can be difficult to study since they may be less open than younger men about their sexual orientation (Kelly, 1977; Kimmel, 1980). However, a few small-scale studies have included a focus on the sexual practices of older gay men (Francher & Henkin, 1972; Kelly, 1977; Kimmel, 1980; Minnigerode & Adelman, 1978). This work has documented one difference between older and younger gay men: the older men appear less likely to frequent "tea rooms" for hidden homosexual encounters (Kelly, 1977). This finding may imply that older gays are less often involved in anonymous sexual situations than are younger gays. Indeed, the number of men in primary sexual relationships has been observed to increase until age 55 (Kelly, 1977). However, after age 55 primary relationships decreased, because of death of a loved one or rejection of the idea of a lifelong lover (Kelly, 1977). Moreover, it is unclear whether the primary sexual relationships in Kelly's study were monogamous or sexually open. Among older people in the San Francisco Behavioral Cohort study (McKusick, Hortsman, & Coates, 1985), only 26% were in monogamous relationships. However, it should be noted that this sample was selected to overrepresent men from environments supporting high-risk sexual behavior (bathhouses, pick-up bars; McKusick, Hortsman, & Coates, 1985). In short, older gays clearly vary between monogamous and nonmonogamous sexual behavior, and there is little evidence to show which type predominates.

Past studies show that most older gay men continue to be sexually active, though the frequency of contacts may decrease with age (Francher & Henkin, 1972; Kelly, 1977; Kimmel, 1980; Minnigerode & Adelman, 1978). However, as with heterosexuals, we still know little about the specifics of the sexual practices of older gays. Since gay men continue to comprise the largest HIV risk category, major effort is needed to determine their current sexual patterns. Because older gays, in contrast to younger ones, may be less "connected" to the gay community, it cannot be assumed that their sexual behavior has paralleled the reductions observed in high-risk sexual activities of younger gays (for reviews see Coates et al., in press; Fineberg, 1988; McKusick, Hortsman, & Coates, 1985).

A CONCEPTUAL MODEL OF AIDS RISK REDUCTION

The research cited in the above sections of this chapter, as well as most research on AIDS and sexual behavior generally, has been atheoretical. Accordingly, in order to improve understanding of risk reduction as it may prevent the wider spread of the epidemic, we have developed the "AIDS Risk Reduction Model (ARRM)" (Catania, Coates, Kegeles, et al., in press; Coates & Greenblatt, 1988). ARRM is a conceptual framework that specifies the processes whereby an individual engaged in high-risk sexual behaviors can change (or fail to change) these behaviors. The model builds on a number of existing models and theories of health behavior change, including the health belief model (Becker, 1974; Janz & Becker, 1984; Maiman & Becker, 1974); self-efficacy theory (Bandura, 1977); diffusion theory (Rogers, 1983); help-seeking models (Fischer, Winer, & Abramowitz, 1983; Gross & McMullen, 1983) and decision-making models (Fishbein & Ajzen, 1975). (Compare the conceptual model of the course of the AIDS disease as an "illness career" presented in the chapter by McKinlay in this volume.)

Our hope for the ARRM is that it will be useful in organizing and interpreting the findings of previous research and in defining directions for research on ways in which individuals at risk for HIV can reduce their risk. We describe ARRM in this chapter as it may be applicable in particular to risk reduction among people at the middle and later ages. We begin with an overview of the model, outlining the stages in the process of risk reduction and the conditions that influence the outcomes at each stage. Then we elaborate on a few selected elements in the model.

Stages in the Processes of Risk Reduction

Figure 5.1 is a schematic diagram of the change processes that relate to possible actions that can reduce the risk of contracting HIV through sexual behavior. These processes are broken into three main stages, as indicated by the diamonds in Figure 5.1. At each of these stages, the individual has the option of taking no action or of taking action that then propels him/her to the next stage. The three stages are: (1) recognizing and labeling one's sexual behavior as high risk for contracting HIV; (2) making a commitment to reduce high-risk sexual contacts and increase low-risk activities; and (3) seeking and enacting strategies to obtain these goals. In brief, ARRM posits that to avoid HIV infection people exhibiting high-risk activities must (1) perceive that their sexual behaviors are placing them at risk for HIV infection—the process referred to as labeling. Then (2) they must be willing to make a strong commitment to changing these activities; this may require deciding whether the behaviors can be altered and whether the benefits of change outweigh the costs. Stage (3) involves enactment of the change, which in turn may require that they be willing to seek help from others in order to obtain solutions. Multiple attempts at seeking solutions through self-help, informal social support, and professional helpers are often needed before an individual achieves the goal of sustaining low-risk behavior (Catania, Pollack, McDermott, Qualls

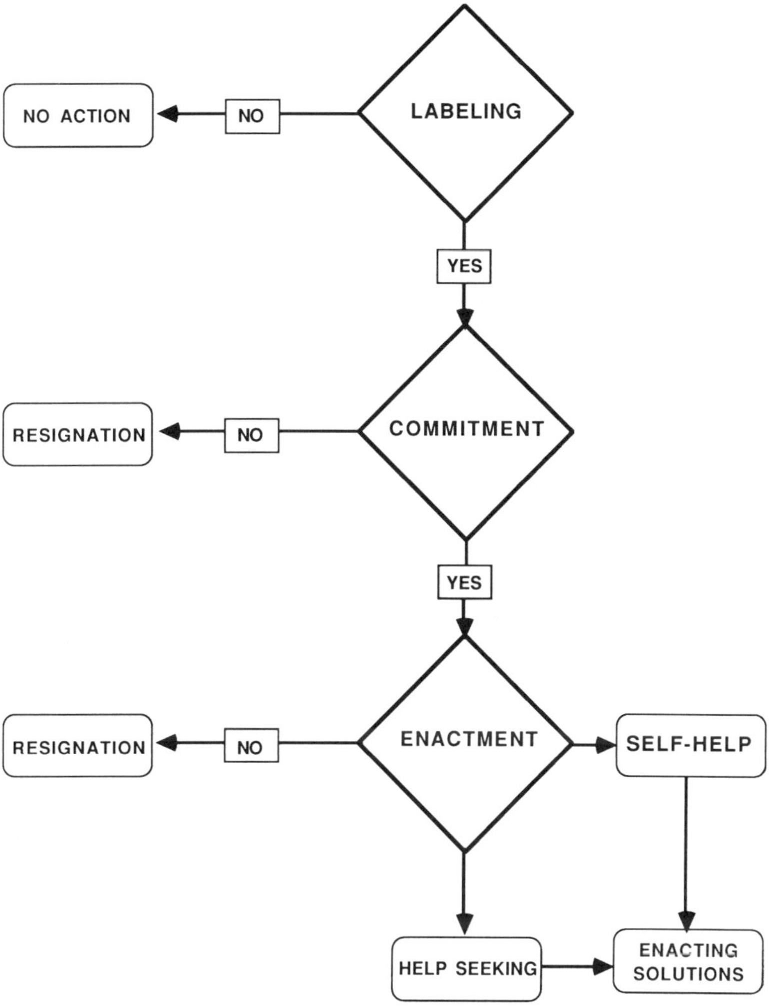

FIGURE 5.1 Stages in the process of risk reduction.

& Cole, in press). In addition, the process of enactment may require complex negotiations with one's sexual partner(s), who may not have achieved the same degree of commitment to pursuing change.

At each stage the processes of labeling, commitment, and enactment are not necessarily either unidirectional or nonreversible. For instance, some individuals may face great difficulty in changing their behavior and come to relabel their activities as nonproblematic, or they may reduce their commitment to change. Additionally, the hypothesized stages may not be invariant. For example, some compliant individuals may not recognize and label their behavior as problematic and bypass the stage of commitment, yet come to change their activities (enactment) because of the urgings of a highly motivated sexual partner.

Influences on Stage Outcomes

Figure 5.2 lists a number of hypothesized cognitive, emotional, and social influences that may affect behavior change at each stage. The column headed "outcome indicators" gives examples of general questions that might be asked in an interview in order to operationalize the possible outcomes. (For elaboration, see Catania, Kegeles, & Coates, in review.) As one example, at the second stage of commitment, change in a person's willingness to use condoms (outcome) can be influenced by his/her perceptions of the impact of condoms on sexual enjoyment and by beliefs concerning condom effectiveness in reducing the risk of disease. Measurement of commitment to using condoms may involve asking how often he/she expects to use condoms during intercourse over the next 4 weeks. Many of the relationships hypothesized by ARRM are supported by research on both gays and heterosexuals, and although this research is not based on older populations, it seems likely that any age differences in risk reduction may be a matter of degree rather than the result of differences in the type of influences operating on this process.

Noted only at Stage 3 in Figure 5.2—although they operate through all three stages—are social networks and group norms. The diffusion of new ideas (e.g., safe sex) throughout a community has been found to depend on social networks and norms that facilitate acceptance of new ideas or behaviors (Rogers, 1983). For health behaviors, social networks and norms have been shown to function in a variety of ways: they may guide the labeling of health problems by influencing health knowledge (Berkman, 1985; Gross & McMullen, 1983; Kaplan, Johnson, Bailey, & Simon, 1987) may channel people toward an appropriate health decision (Berkman, 1985); or may influence health-relevant beliefs (e.g., self-efficacy beliefs). Among heterosexuals, group norms have been shown to influence contraceptive behavior (Condelli, 1986; Nathanson & Becker, 1986). Studies of young gay respondents have shown that the degree of social support and strength of group norms prescribing safe sex practices are inversely related both to the frequency of unprotected receptive anal intercourse (San Francisco AIDS Foundation, 1987) and to the number of sex partners (Emmons, Joseph, Kessler, et al., 1986; Richardson, Schott, McGuigan, & Levine, 1987); in addition, these group influences predict avoidance of anonymous sex partners (Joseph, Montgomery, Emmons, et al., 1987). (Some of these

Stage	*Some [Hypothesized] Influences*	*Outcome Indicators*
One : Labeling	*Susceptibility* *Trans. Know.* *Aversive Emotions*	Is your sexual behavior putting you at risk for HIV infection?
Two : Commitment	*Aversive Emotions* *Perceptions of:* *enjoyment* *risk reduction* *Self-Efficacy* *Condom Attitudes*	Do you expect to do "x" in the next 4 weeks?
Three : Enactment	*Aversive Emotions* *Communication* *Primary* *New Partners* *Informal Networking* *Formal Help-Seeking*	What have you done?

General Model

Enactment = Stage 3 Influences + Commitment + Labeling

FIGURE 5.2 AIDS Risk Reduction Model Influences

findings have been disputed by Emmons, Joseph, Kessler, et al., 1986; and Joseph, Montgomery, Emmons, et al., 1987.) Conversely, social networks may inhibit labeling high-risk behaviors as a problem, as through social stigmatization (Fischer, Winer, & Abramowitz, 1983).

Help-Seeking Behavior

The AIDS Risk Reduction Model posits that (at Stage 3) seeking help from either informal or formal sources is a major social pathway by which people initiate and reinforce changes in high-risk sexual behavior (Catania, Coates, Kegeles, et al., in press; Catania, Kegeles, & Coates, 1988). As a heuristic guide to HIV prevention, the model postulates that individual help-seeking is an integral part of solving an essentially social problem. The first step in initiating safe sex (enactment) is often through seeking the assistance of one's sexual partner in meeting this goal. Obviously, verbal communication and problem-solving skills are needed to engage one's partner successfully in safe sex behavior. Interestingly, Catania (in press) has found that sexual communication skills may be less developed among members of older people than younger ones, indicating that some older individuals may need training in these social skills if they are to adopt safe sex practices in a successful fashion.

Help-seeking is also a process by which people may contact formal prevention programs. As such, it may facilitate the diffusion of intervention effects throughout a community (Rogers, 1983). Previous research suggests that if a large segment of a community seeks help with addressing safe sex issues, there will be a rapid diffusion of innovations directed at reducing HIV risk. Moreover, people seeking help themselves may in turn contribute to the formal program by serving as lay helpers to others who seek it. For community-based interventions to be successful, then, they may need to identify and train the existing sources of help in a community as well as creating new sources of aid.

When older people are the help-seekers, the model points to the importance of understanding their existing patterns of help-seeking and the determinants of possible changes in these patterns. Several relevant studies have shown that help-seeking behaviors vary by age, although it is not always clear whether this represents an aging or cohort phenomenon (Veroff, Kulka, & Douvan, 1981; Waxman, Carner, & Klein, 1984). These studies indicate that use of mental health services declines with age (Veroff, Kulka, & Douvan, 1981; Waxman, Carner, & Klein, 1984). A slight increase in professional usage is evident among middle-aged males (Veroff, Kulka, & Douvan, 1981), which may reflect the greater monetary resources possessed by that group (Veroff, Kulka, & Douvan, 1981). Earlier studies show that while older people use fewer formal services, especially for marital problems, they utilize more self-help strategies than younger people (Pearlin & Schooler, 1978). More recent studies indicate that young adults exhibit more informal support seeking than middle-aged or older adults (Irion & Blanchard-Fields, 1987). The generalizability of these findings to older people facing problems with reducing high-risk sexual practices is uncertain. However, from the perspective of diffusion theory, older people's help-seeking patterns may inhibit rapid dissemination of AIDS-relevant knowledge among this age category. This possibility raises serious concerns about the usefulness of community-level interventions for older persons. (See the chapters in this volume by McKinlay and Crystal, respectively.)

A RESEARCH AGENDA FOR PRIMARY PREVENTION

Several areas of needed research are brought to attention by the AIDS Risk Reduction Model. There is a particular need to generate a knowledge base for developing and targeting primary preventions for older individuals and couples.

The model is useful not only for defining such research areas, but also in piecing together existing psychosocial findings.

First, and fundamental to prevention research, is the need for a sound data base on the prevalence and distribution of HIV infection in the older population. Is HIV distributed randomly or is it clustered in particular segments of this population? The answer to this question has important implications for efforts to target groups for intervention. In addition, there is a need to identify the conditions under which older persons will seek HIV antibody testing—an important element in primary prevention efforts (Coates, Morin, Lo, et al., 1987). Testing is also important to secondary prevention efforts, because knowing that one is HIV-positive may lead to closer monitoring of one's health and, possibly, to earlier detection and treatment of opportunistic infections. It is important, then, to ascertain how older people might be motivated and enabled to seek HIV testing and to define the conditions that prevent test-seeking by those who might otherwise obtain it. For example, are economic conditions or transportation problems impeding older persons who seek testing?

A second area needing investigation relates to older people's knowledge and beliefs about AIDS. Prior studies have demonstrated the importance of knowledge and belief systems in influencing high-risk behavior (for review see Catania, Kegeles, & Coates, in review; Coates et al., in press). Yet a recent national survey ($n = 885$) indicated that 43% of older Americans (50+ years), compared to 24% of younger respondents, had never heard of the HIV antibody test (Dawson, Cynamon, & Fitti, 1987). Understanding such gaps in older people's knowledge is clearly vital to informing and motivating them to engage in appropriate behaviors.

A third research need is for behavioral studies to identify the prevalence and characteristics within the older population of those engaged in high-risk sexual activities. In addition, what social conditions lead to high-risk behavior among older people? What types of interventions and methods of delivery would best serve the diverse segments of the older American population? Prior research indicates that certain older individuals will seek out sex education and therapy and will learn to change their sexual behavior, beliefs, and knowledge regarding sexual matters (for reviews see Bonner, Gendel, Catania, & Pollack, 1986; White & Catania, 1982). However, little is known about those other older people with sexual problems or concerns who never seek professional help (Catania, in press). Research also indicates that community-based interventions that target well-defined communities may be particularly useful for large-scale intervention purposes (Catania, Coates, Kegeles, et al., in press; Coates & Greenblatt, 1988; Coates, Stall, Catania, Dolcini & Hoff, in press), but the categories of older people at risk for HIV infection must be more clearly defined. Clearer understanding is needed of both the informal and formal help sources older people utilize with respect to sexual issues and the types of new "helpers" that would be acceptable to given communities of older people (cf.

Catania, Coates, Kegeles, et al., in press). Among other goals, AIDS interventions need to focus on changing sexual behavior in ways that facilitate a satisfying continuation of older people's sex lives and need to be tailored to the physiological diversity in this population.

SOME SUMMARY NOTES

This chapter has emphasized that, contrary to much widespread opinion, AIDS is a disease that has permeated all facets of society. It is not exclusively a white gay male disease, nor is it exclusively a disease of the young. Middle-aged and elderly people are dying of AIDS and in all likelihood are continuing to transmit HIV to those they love. The transmission processes outlined in our review suggest that older Americans are or will be experiencing a significant—if perhaps limited—increase in HIV infection over the next 5 to 10 years. However, until more systematic research is conducted on the sexual practices of older heterosexual, bisexual, and gay individuals, the limits of HIV transmission in these populations cannot be defined. Our proposed research agenda suggests the knowledge needed for intervening with older people at risk for HIV infection and for identifying who in the older population should be targeted for intervention. This agenda also includes work needed to assess older people's perceptions of acceptable sources of help for AIDS-related concerns.

In particular, we have outlined a model, ARRM, that provides a conceptual framework for organizing existing findings and guiding future research on risk reduction in middle and old age. This model calls for identifying the specific conditions with respect to older people that facilitate or inhibit: (1) correct labeling of HIV risk behaviors, (2) making commitments to change risk behaviors, and (3) successful enactment of strategies to reduce high-risk behaviors.

REFERENCES

Anderson, K., B. Gorgone, R. Marlink, R. Ferriani, M. Essex, P. Benz, and J. Groopman. 1986. "Transfusion Acquired HIV Infection among Immunocompromised Persons." *Annals of Internal Medicine* 105:519–527.

Bandura, A. 1977. "Self-Efficacy: Toward a Unifying Theory of Behavioral Change." *Psychological Review* 84:191–215.

Becker, M.H. 1974. "The Health Belief Model and Personal Health Behavior." *Health Education Monographs* 2:220–243.

Berezin, M. 1976. "Sex and Old Age: A Further Review of the Literature." *Journal of Geriatric Psychiatry* 9:189–209.

Berglund, O., S. Beckman, L. Grillner, B. Jansson, P. Lidbrink, A. Karlsson, L. Morfeldt-Mansson, P. Pehrson, M. Torngren, B. Wiechel, and O. Akerblom. 1988. "HIV Transmission by Blood Transfusions in Stockholm 1979–1985." *AIDS* 2:51–54.

Berkman, L. 1985. "The Relationship of Social Networks and Social Support to Morbidity and Mortality." Pp. 241–262 in *Social Support and Health,* edited by S. Cohen and S. Syme. New York: Academic Press.

Bonner, E., E. Gendel, J. Catania, and L. Pollack. 1986. *Reasons for Terminating Sex Therapy among Older Clients.* Paper presented at the Gerontological Society of America meetings, Chicago, IL. Paper available from J. Catania.

Catania, J. in press. "Help-Seeking Associated with Sexual Problems: An Avenue for Adult Sexual Development." *Dissertation Abstracts International.*

Catania, J., S. Kegeles, S., and T. Coates. in review. "Towards an Understanding of Risk Behavior: An AIDS Risk Reduction Model (ARRM)." Paper available from the first author.

Catania, J., S. Kegeles, and T. Coates. 1988. *Seeking Help for Problems in Reducing High Risk Sexual Behavior.* IV International Conference on AIDS, Stockholm, Sweden.

Catania, J., T. Coates, S. Kegeles, M. Extrant, J. Guydish, and L. Bye. in press. "Implications of the AIDS Risk Reduction Model for the Gay Community: The Importance of Perceived Sexual Enjoyment and Help-Seeking Behaviors." In *Psychological approaches to the prevention of AIDS (VCPP),* edited by G. Albee and V. Mays. Hanover and London: University Press of New England.

Coates, T., and R. Greenblatt. 1988. "Behavioral Change Using Interventions at the Community Level." In *Sexually Transmitted Diseases,* edited by M.K. Holmes et al. New York: McGraw Hill.

Coates, T., S. Morin, B. Lo, R. Stall, and L. McKusick. 1987. *AIDS Antibody Testing: Will It Stop the AIDS Epidemic? Will It Help People Infected with HIV?* Invited address, American Psychological Association Meetings, New York.

Coates, T., R. Stall, J. Catania, P. Dolcini, and C. Hoff. in press. "Prevention of HIV Infection in High Risk Groups." In *1988 AIDS Clinical Review,* edited by P. Volberding and M. Jacobson. New York: Marcel Dekker.

Condelli, L. 1986. "Social and Attitudinal Determinants of Contraceptive Choice: Using the Health Belief Model." *The Journal of Sex Research* 22:478–491.

Curran, J., H. Jaffe, A. Hardy, W. Morgan, R. Selik, and T. Dondero. 1988. "Epidemiology of HIV Infection and AIDS in the United States." *Science* 239:610–616.

Dawson, D., M. Cynamon, and J. Fitti. 1987. "AIDS Knowledge and Attitudes: Provisional Data from the National Health Interview Survey United States, August, (1987)." *Advance Data,* Vital and Health Satistics of the National Center for Health Statistics, Department of Health and Human Services, Number 146, November 19.

Downey, L. 1980. "Intergenerational Change in Sex Behavior: A Belated Look at Kinsey's Males." *Archives of Sexual Behavior* 9:267–317.

Dressel, P., and W. Avant. 1983. "Range of Alternatives." P. 201 in *Sexuality In the Later Years: Roles and Behavior,* edited by R. Weg. New York: Academic Press.

Emmons, C., J. Joseph, R. Kessler, C. Wortman, S. Montgomery, and D. Ostrow. 1986. "Psychosocial Predictors of Reported Behavior Change in Homosexual Men at Risk for AIDS." *Health Education Quarterly* 13:331–345.

Felstein, I. 1983. "Dysfunction: Origins and Therapeutic Approaches." P. 234 in *Sexuality In the Later Years: Roles and Behavior,* edited by R. Weg. New York: Academic Press.

Fineberg, H. 1988. "Education to Prevent AIDS: Prospects and Obstacles." *Science* 239:592–596.

Fishbein, M., and I. Ajzen. 1975. *Belief, Attitude, Intention, and Behavior: An Introduction to Theory and Research.* Reading, MA: Addison-Wesley.

Fischer, E., D. Winer, and S. Abramowitz. 1983. "Seeking Professional Help for Psychological Problems." In *New Directions in Helping: Applied Perspectives on Help Seeking and Receiving,* Vol. 3, edited by A. Nadler, J. Fisher, and B. DePaulo. New York: Academic Press.

Francher, J., and J. Henkin. 1972. "The Menopausal Queen: Adjustment to Aging and the Male Homosexual." *American Journal of Orthopsychiatry* 43:670–674.

Friedman, B., T. Burns, and M. Schork. 1980. *A Study of National Trends in Transfusion Practice.* Report to the National Heart Lung and Blood Institute. National Technical Information Service PB81-125437.

Gross, A., and P. McMullen. 1983. "Models of the Help Seeking Process." In *New Directions in Helping: Help Seeking,* Vol. 2, edited by B. DePaulo, A. Nadler, and J. Fisher. New York: Academic Press.

Irion, J., and F. Blanchard-Fields. 1987. "A Cross-Sectional Comparison of Adaptive Coping in Adulthood." *Journal of Gerontology* 42:502–504.

Janz, N.K., and M.H. Becker. 1984. "The Health Belief Model: A Decade Later." *Health Education Quarterly* 11:1–47.

Joseph, J., S. Montgomery, C. Emmons, R. Kessler, D. Ostrow, C. Wortman, M. O'Brien, and S. Eshleman. 1987. "Magnitude and Determinants of Behavioral Risk Reduction: Longitudinal Analysis of a Cohort at Risk for AIDS." *Psychology and Health* 1:73–96.

Kalbfleisch, J., and J. Lawless. 1988. *A Comment on Estimation of Incubation Periods and Epidemic Parameters Based on Data on AIDS Patients Infected by Blood Transfusion.* Technical Report Series STAT-87-24, University of Waterloo, Department of Statistics and Actuaral Science, Canada.

Kaplan, H., R. Johnson, C. Bailey, and W. Simon. 1987. "The Sociological Study of AIDS: A Critical Review of the Literature and Suggested Research Agenda." *Journal of Health and Social Behavior* 28:140–157.

Kelly, J. 1977. "The Aging Male Homosexual." *Gerontologist* 17:328–332.

Kimmel, D. 1980. "Life-History Interviews of Aging Gay Men." *International Journal of Aging and Human Development* 10:239–248.

L'age-Stehr, J., A. Schwarz, G. Offerman, J.H. Langmaack, I. Bennhold, M. Niedrig, and M. Koch. 1985. "HTLV-III in Kidney Transplant Recipients." *The Lancet* (December): 1361–1362.

Lifson, A. 1988. "Do Alternate Modes for Transmission of HIV Exist?: A Review." *Journal of the American Medical Association* 259:1353–1356.

Ludeman, K. 1981. "The Sexuality of the Older Person: Review of the Literature." *Gerontologist* 21:203–208.

Maiman, L.A., and M.H. Becker. 1974. "The Health Belief Model: Origins and Correlates in Psychological Theory." *Health Education Monographs* 2:336–353.

Makinodan, T. 1977. "Immunity and Aging." Pp. 384–387 in *Handbook of The Biology of Aging,* edited by C. Finch and L. Hayflick. New York: Van Nostrand Reinhold Co.

Martin, C. 1975. "Marital and Sexual Factors in Relation to Age, Disease and Longevity." Pp. 326–347 in *Life History Research in Psychopathology,* Vol. 4, edited by R. Wirt, G. Winokur, and M. Roff. Minneapolis, Minn: University of Minnesota Press.

McKusick, L., W. Hortsman, and T. Coates. 1985. "AIDS and the Sexual Behavior Reported by Gay Men in San Francisco." *American Journal of Public Health* 75:493–496.

Menitove, J. 1986. "Status of Recipients of Blood from Donors Subsequently Found to Have Antibody to HIV." *New England Journal of Medicine* 315:1095–1096.

Minnigerode, F., and M. Adelman. 1978. "Elderly Homosexual Women and Men: Report on a Pilot Study." *The Family Coordinator* 27:451–456.

Nathanson, C., and M. Becker. 1986. "Family and Peer Influence on Obtaining a Method of Contraception." *Journal of Marriage and the Family* 48:513–525.

National Academy of Sciences, Institute of Medicine. 1986. *Confronting AIDS: Directions for Public Health, Health Care, and Research,* p. 60.

Padian, N., L. Marquis, D. Francis, R. Anderson, G. Rutherford, P. O'Malley, and W. Winkelstein. 1987. "Male-to-Female Transmission of HIV." *Journal of the American Medical Association* 258:790–798.

Pearlin, L., and C. Schooler. 1978. "The Structure of Coping." *Journal of Health and Social Behavior* 19:2–21.

Peterman, T., H. Jaffe, P. Feorino, J. Getchell, D. Warfield, H. Haverkos, R. Stoneburner, and J. Curran. 1985. "Transfusion-Associated AIDS in the United States." *Journal of the American Medical Association* 254:2913–2917.

Peterman, T., K. Lui, D. Lawrence, and J. Allen. 1987. "Estimating the Risk of Transfusion-Associated AIDS and HIV Infection." *Transfusion* 27:371–374.

Peterman, T., R. Stoneburner, J. Allen, H. Jaffe, and J. Curran. 1988. "Risk of HIV Transmission from Heterosexual Adults with Transfusion-Associated Infections." *Journal of the American Medical Association* 259:55–58.

Pfeiffer, E., A. Verwoerdt, and G. Davis. 1972. "Sexual Behavior in Middle Life." *American Journal of Psychiatry* 128:1262–1267.

Piot, P., J. Kreiss, J. Ndinya-Achola, E. Ngugi, J. Simonsen, D. Cameron, H. Tailman, and F. Plummer. 1987. "Heterosexual Transmission of HIV." *AIDS* 1:199–206.

Richardson, J., J. Schott, K. McGuigan, and A. Levine. 1987. "Behavior Change among Homosexual College Students to Decrease Risk for Acquired Immune Deficiency Syndrome." *Preventive Medicine* 16:285–286.

Rogers, E.M. 1983. *Diffusion of Innovation.* New York: Free Press.

San Francisco AIDS Foundation. 1987. "Designing an Effective AIDS Risk Prevention Campaign Strategy for San Francisco: Results from the Fourth Probability Sample of an Urban Gay Male Community." San Francisco, CA: Research Decision Corporation, Communication Technologies.

Schlesinger, B. 1983. "Institutional Life: The Canadian Experience." P. 262 in *Sexuality In the Later Years: Roles and Behavior,* edited by R. Weg. New York: Academic Press.

Veroff, J., R. Kulka, and E. Douvan. 1981. *Mental Health in America: Patterns of Help Seeking from 1957 to 1976.* New York: Basic Books.

Ward, J., D. Deppe, S. Samson, H. Perkins, P. Holland, L. Fernando, P. Feorino, P. Thompsons, S. Kleinman, and J. Allen. 1987. "Risk of HIV Infection from Blood Donors Who Later Developed AIDS." *Annals of Internal Medicine* 106:61–62.

Waxman, H., E. Carner, and M. Klein. 1984. "Underutilization of Mental Health Professionals by Community Elderly." *Gerontologist* 24:23–30.

Weg, R. 1978. "The Physiology of Sex and Aging." In *Sexuality and Aging,* edited by R. Solnick. Los Angeles: University of Southern California Press.

Weg, R. 1983. "The Physiological Perspective." In *Sexuality In the Later Years: Roles and Behavior,* edited by R. Weg. New York: Academic Press.

White, C., and J. Catania. 1982. "Psychoeducational Intervention for Sexuality with the Aged, Family Members of the Aged and People Who Work with the Aged." *International Journal of Aging and Human Development* 15:121–138.

CHAPTER 6

Methodological Considerations in Research on Sexual Behavior and AIDS among Older People

Judith A. Levy and Gary L. Albrecht

This chapter, which focuses on AIDS as a special case, examines some of the methodological problems of conducting research on the sexual knowledge, attitudes, and behavior of older Americans and examines strategies for handling these difficulties. As emphasized throughout this book, such research is important because there is little definitive knowledge about human sexual activity and attitudes in general, and even less about that of older Americans (Weg, 1983). Moreover, concern about the spread of AIDS and other sexually transmitted diseases to individuals of all ages forces us to assess the relative risk and general impact of AIDS on older people and hence, by definition, to examine their sexual behavior.

At first glance, the study of sexual behavior among older Americans may not appear interesting or fruitful because of widespread beliefs that when reproduction has ended sexual activity and number of sexual partners must diminish, and that the threat of older people contracting AIDS or other sexually transmitted diseases (STDs) must be small. Consequently, there has been little impetus to study sexual behavior or AIDS and sexually transmitted diseases in late adulthood. On the contrary, however, there is scattered evidence that many older Americans remain sexually active into their eighties, some have multiple partners, and a full range of sexual behaviors are practiced (Lee, 1987; Starr & Weiner, 1981). Rather than relying on untested assumptions and potentially fallacious conventional wisdom, solid research is needed to extend our understanding of sexual attitudes and

The authors received support from the National Institute on Aging to write this paper. They wish to thank Matilda White Riley, Marcia Ory, Diane Zablotsky, and the members of the NIA AIDS Advisory Group for their comments on this work.

behaviors at all stages of the life course, including late adulthood. As part of this research effort, studies are needed that identify the epidemiology, risks, and effective health promotion programs concerning AIDS and the spread of sexually transmitted diseases for our older population.

Based on the need for such work, this chapter discusses inherent methodological problems and illustrates strategies for conducting research on the sexual behavior of older Americans with a particular emphasis on AIDS. First, we discuss the special types of populations to be studied and the selection of units of analysis. Then we consider the issues of sampling and data collection procedures and instruments. As special threats to validity in research on sex and AIDS, we discuss refusals and missing values. Finally, we present the ethical dilemmas of sex and AIDS research, including problems related to maintaining study confidentiality and obtaining the subject's informed consent.

The objective throughout is to show how well-established principles of social science research need to be emphasized, adapted, or specified when the focus of investigation is on both highly sensitive subject matter and older people—not only as individuals, but also as partners in intimate personal relationships. Although its content spans the social sciences, sex research often ignores many of the theoretical insights or methodological principles that these disciplines offer (Bentler & Abramson, 1981). Perhaps this disregard for standard scientific knowledge and practices is traceable to the marginal status of sex research in general. Nonetheless, the reliability, validity, and utility of sex studies would be improved through better use of existing social science theories and techniques (Lee, 1987). Also, human sexuality involves both biological and social processes (Butler & Lewis, 1976), and greater interdisciplinary collaboration between the biological and social sciences would prove profitable. Such collaboration is particularly critical in the study of AIDS. For example, there are many indications that life stress may contribute to immune suppression in the host and thus increase susceptibility to the AIDS virus and its associated outcomes (Kaplan et al., 1987; Livingston, 1988). Understanding the process and risk for seroconversion in people exposed to the AIDS virus requires exploration of both biological and social factors. (See the chapter by Maddox and Maddox in this volume.)

STUDY POPULATIONS AND UNITS OF ANALYSIS

In studies of sexual behavior or of AIDS, the choice of populations to be sampled as well as the unit of analysis depends upon the particular research objective. When investigating the sexual activities and AIDS-related behaviors of older people, the appropriate unit of analysis might be, for example, individuals in the general population, members of cohorts born at a particular time or undergoing a particular experience, persons at high risk (such as sexually active gay men or frequently transfused hemophiliacs), women over 70, those with diverse racial/ethnic backgrounds, or those who vote. With very different implications, the unit of analysis may be groups rather than individuals, such as sexual dyads, extended family and social networks, or those who vote. Selection of the unit of analysis will affect the design of the study and the conclusions that can be drawn from the data.

The Life Course and Social Networks

Two conceptual approaches are especially important to the choice of study populations and research units, as well as to every other aspect of research design: the life-course approach and the network approach.[1] The life-course perspective has provided new insight into the occurrence, timing, and sequencing of events and transitions that mark movement across life from birth to death (Hogan, 1980; Riley, 1985). Within the context of individual lives, people undertake multiple "careers" or trajectories that include work, family, and sexual conduct (Elder, 1985). These careers are interconnected at a personal level and also intersect with the career paths of others. Indeed, the occurrence and frequency of sexual activity in the later years appear to be influenced more by the availability of partners than age-related biological decline (Comfort, 1976; Starr & Weiner, 1981; Starr, 1985). Therefore, understanding of sexual beliefs and conduct during the later years often requires information on life-course patterns of respondents and on how such patterns interact with the life events and life-course transitions of significant others.

Similarly, the research at hand requires understanding of social networks. Until recently, older Americans often were popularly conceptualized erroneously as a socially isolated, dependent, and homogeneous subgroup, removed from the mainstream of society. These assumptions have been widely challenged through scientific research, and it is now clearly demonstrated that a variety of interactional patterns, activities, beliefs, and life events characterize the later years of the life course (for a summary, see Hagestad & Neugarten, 1985). With the extension of longevity in postindustrial society, older persons comprise an increasingly larger and potentially more powerful segment of the total population. For example, as evidenced by the activities of groups such as the American Association of Retired Persons,

[1] Discussion of these approaches has profited from the incisive and detailed discussion of network analysis and the life-course perspective applied to the study of human sexual behavior in the 1987 technical proposal of the National Opinion Research Center, "Social and Behavioral Aspects of Health and Fertility Related Behavior."

older Americans have the potential to become one of the strongest emergent political action and lobby groups in the country. Retail companies are concentrating on them as one of the leading markets in the next decade. Furthermore, older people are embedded in many complex social networks in the community that revolve around three- and four-generation families, churches, residences, service organizations, clubs, investment organizations, and community groups. There is continuity and embeddedness in the lives of older people that can only be apprehended in both a life-course and a social network perspective.

Types of Networks

Networks that pertain to the study of sexual behavior and AIDS among older people include the following four types: The first are the networks of current and past sexual contacts that may effect exposure to the HIV virus. The second is the network of blood donations and transfusions that allows exposure to the virus through a tainted blood supply. This type of network is extremely sensitive to timing and sequencing because of changes in the nature and extent of screening of blood supplies. The third involves information networks that characterize the flow of communications about AIDS to older people and from older people to others. The fourth type consists of political action networks of older Americans concerned with AIDS issues.

The sexual contact and blood donation/transfusion networks reflect the individual's social world and relationships that can account for directly contracting AIDS. The information and political action networks indirectly bear on the AIDS problem by examining the diffusion of information and shaping of social policies.

SAMPLING

Drawing a representative sample is one of the more challenging and typically least successful aspects of sex research (for an early discussion, see George & Weiler, 1981).

Sampling Older People

Sampling techniques for general population studies of older adults' knowledge, attitudes, and sexual behavior must be sensitive to the fact that older people are located in a wide range of households and living arrangements such as single-family dwellings, nursing homes, hospices or long-term care facilities, retirement homes and villages, trailer parks, and homes of adult offspring.

Consideration also must be given to "snow birds," as numerous elderly migrate to accommodate the weather during the year. Because women outnumber men in the older age strata, special care must be taken to ensure a representative subsample of men.

Sampling People at Risk

In AIDS research, a sampling of older people at risk for the virus can include those who received blood transfusions prior to effective screening, homosexuals, bisexuals, and former and/or present IV drug abusers as well as their sex partners. Where sexual behavior is a primary focus, appropriate means must be found for sampling sexual dyads rather than individuals. In studies where transmission of the AIDS virus is of primary interest, social nodes of sexual contact may be more important than coupled acts. For example, studies of disease transmission among gay men might include a network analysis of gay bars, bathhouses, and private clubs. Similarly, drug networks and other social units may be more important than individuals in studies of AIDS among illegal drug users and their sexual partners. Such networks tend to be differentiated on the basis of community location, demographic characteristics, and patterns of drug use (see Wiebel, 1987). Tracing of interactional patterns can also involve sexual contacts made during international travel and sexual exposure to men living in cities with high prevalence rates for the virus (Darrow, Gorman, & Glick, 1986a). A reconstructed scenario in Norway, for instance, retrospectively documents how a Norwegian sailor brought the HIV virus home to his wife from Africa in 1966. The sailor, his wife, and daughter born in 1967 all died of AIDS in 1976. Two daughters born before 1967 show no signs of AIDS and test negative for AIDS antibodies (Van, 1988). Such examples highlight the practical utility of using social networks as sampling frames.

Sampling People with AIDS

Drawing a representative sample of people who have AIDS or those infected with the AIDS virus is complicated by the problem of determining who fits the medical criteria (Siegel & Bauman, 1986). Tests for seropositivity often report inaccurate results, and individuals who initially test negative may be in an incubationary period. Although a case definition for AIDS has been developed by the Centers for Disease Control (CDC), symptoms of the disease vary widely and physicians differ considerably in their judgments. Moreover, CDC has continued to revise its criteria as new findings and information become available (Zich & Temoshok, 1986). Thus, research designs based upon repeated sampling potentially risk sampling individuals at the end of the study whose characteristics differ from the criteria that governed selection of the sample when the study began. Such shifting definitions limit the comparability of research findings at different points in time.

In addition to problems related to ambiguous criteria, sampling problems also arise when people hide or deny having AIDS or conceal their high-risk behaviors to avoid negative consequences. Reluctance about disclosure is reinforced by the social stigma attached to many of the transmittal routes for the virus (Albert, 1986; Callero et al., 1986; Conrad, 1986; and see the chapter in this book by McKinlay). For example, IV drug abuse and prostitution are punishable by law, a circumstance unlikely to encourage open disclosure about these activities. Meanwhile, people who are homosexual or bisexual may prefer not to have their sexual preferences or behavior known because they fear discrimination and retribution (National Gay and Lesbian Task Force, 1988). Even people who contract the disease through blood transfusions are not immune to public censorship (Dawson et al., 1987; NCHS, 1987).

Handling Sampling Problems

Despite these difficulties, samples of infected, stigmatized, or reluctant populations may be gained through various methods. Blood donors or those who have received blood transfusions can be identified through medical records, donor registries, and physician practices (see, for example, Callero et al., 1986). These sources along with hospitals and hospice care facilities also are useful in identifying AIDS cases. Researchers interested in the spread of AIDS among prostitutes and IV drug abusers often gain entry to drug networks through the sponsorship of current and former members. Samples of gay and bisexual men are drawn by placing advertisements in gay periodicals, through appeals to clinic populations, through word of mouth (see, for example, Emmons et al., 1986), or through self-identification (Bye, 1984, 1985). Gay bars, bathhouses, and other gay organizations and establishments are other common sampling frames.

Sample Biases

Samples based on volunteers and self-identified subjects raise serious questions about sample biases. One concern is that volunteers may differ in important ways from others in a population. For example, Wolchik, Braver, and Jensen (1985) compared the characteristics of volunteers to nonvolunteers in a study of sexual experience and attitudes. Findings suggest that men are more likely than women to volunteer, and that volunteers of both sexes are more sexually experienced, report more exposure to erotic materials, and worry less about their sexual performance than nonvolunteers. Meanwhile, Kortarba and Lang (1986) observe that studies of gay communities that recruit samples through gay establishments potentially exclude those men who do not frequent these settings. Snowball sampling techniques, which ask key informants for their help in obtaining a desired sample, can partially offset this problem by locating potential subjects who might not be identified through other means (Siegel & Bauman, 1986). This technique is unlikely, however, to identify those men who are socially isolated or do not associate with a particular network (Welch, 1975).

Weighted Samples

Because research on sex or AIDS is especially likely to rely on small or specialized samples, it often requires the use of sampling weights for analyses. As is true for all research, weights also may be needed to compensate for such critical concerns as the probability of finding people at home, race and ethnic differences in access to telephones, and age and gender differences in availability, given labor force participation (see *Gallup,* 1986). In studies where age differences are a factor, the older the age category, the smaller the potential pool of subjects available for a simple random sample; also, the fewer the number of older men relative to older women.

Often, sampling biases requiring adjustment through the use of sampling weights are not apparent until after the data are collected. In a study of AIDS in Chicago, Albrecht, Levy, and Sugrue (1987), for example, discovered that a random digit dialing procedure used in a telephone survey produced a sample of 41% men and 59% women. Other studies confirm that women are more likely than men to agree to telephone interviews (Kovar & Fitti, 1985).

DATA COLLECTION PROCEDURES

In principle, studies of aging, sex, and AIDS should be able to draw upon the full range of scientific design and data collection methods. In practice, however, most AIDS and sex research rely on some form of self-reported information, as intimate behavior typically takes place in privacy without an audience or formal record. Some exceptions do occur, however. This section will cover experience with some of the more promising methods for collecting data on sex or AIDS among older people, including a discussion of the strengths and drawbacks of each method.

Telephone Surveys and Mail Questionnaires

Telephone surveys, employing random digit dialing procedures, are a cost-effective and reasonably well-developed technique for use with targeted AIDS high-risk groups (see Bye, 1984, 1985), as with the general population. Telephone surveys of sensitive topics are attractive because respondents feel safe, comfortable, and can answer anonymously. They also are less costly than face-to-face interviews (Groves & Kahn, 1979) and work equally well with young or older people (Herzog & Rogers, 1988). The latter often prefer them to direct contact with an interviewer out of fear of being victimized by a stranger. Telephone access to older people also is generally good, since older adults are even more likely than younger people to have a telephone in their household (Thornberry & Massey, 1987, is an early example).

Nonetheless, telephone interviews do pose special drawbacks when used with an elderly sample. On the average, older adults have higher rates of disability and serious illness than younger people in the general population. These health problems can prevent them from answering the phone or talking for extended periods. Also, many older people have weak voices that do not carry or record well on electronic devices (Reinharz & Rowles, 1987). In addition, over 25% of people over age 65 experience some degree of hearing loss (Hagness, 1984), a condition that potentially limits their ability to respond on the phone. Interviewers, however, can offset the effects of hearing loss by speaking slowly and clearly on the phone. Kovar and Fitti (1985), for example, used this technique to obtain a 94.2% response rate for the hearing impaired subsample of an NCHS study. In contrast, they were able to attain only a 92% response rate for the nonimpaired portion of the sample.

Mailed questionnaires offer another data collection strategy, although their use often produces serious sampling biases; for example, questionnaires may be answered by someone other than the person to whom they were addressed —with women more likely than men to act as surrogates in filling out the surveys (Bloch & Nebenzahl, 1983). Combining telephone surveys with mail questionnaires may get around some of the problems, although not without other methodological costs. Brambilla and McKinlay (1987) employed a mixture of mailed questionnaires and telephone interviews in a 1981–82 health survey in Massachusetts. While they received a combined response rate of 77%, they discovered that the two different methods introduced different sample selection biases. These findings emphasize the desirability for social scientists to identify and report information in published articles on who supplied answers to their questions and the circumstances under which data were collected. Such information allows readers to judge the limits and validity of a study's findings.

Self-Administered Questionnaires

Self-administered questionnaires offer a number of advantages in the study of sensitive topics (Siegel & Bauman, 1986). They are economical and they reduce the demands of responding to someone directly, but on the other hand they generally have low response rates and are not suited for gathering couples data. Moreover, unless the the interviewer is present, it is not always certain that the intended respondent is the person who filled out the form. Because of their many strengths, however, self-administered questionnaires have been widely used in AIDS research (see, for example, Emmons et al., 1986; Ginzburg et al., 1986; Martin, 1986; McKusick, Hortsman, & Coates, 1985; Simkins & Kushner, 1986; Stall et al., 1986; Williams, 1986).

Face-to-Face Interviews

Face-to-face interviews, another widely used data collection strategy, offer researchers the advantage of building an empathic relationship with the respondent while exerting partial control over the situation and the setting where the data are collected. Personal interviews can of course be combined with self-administered questionnaires to extend the type and range of information that is collected. Both techniques have proven useful in studies of sex and AIDS (see, for example, Beeson, Zones, & Nye, 1986; Emmons et al., 1986; Joseph, et al., 1987; Martin, 1987), and in gathering information from older adults (Herzog & Rodgers, 1988).

Observational Techniques

Among observational techniques, Humphreys' (1970) classic study of homosexual behavior in the "tea room" trade offers one of the better-known examples of observation of sexual behavior. Masters and Johnson (1966, 1970) also used observational techniques, including medical indicators, in conducting their study of human physiology and sexual response. In AIDS research, at least two studies (Ginzburg et al., 1986; Wiebel, 1987) relied on observational techniques to collect data on drug users and their sexual partners. Lessor and Jurich (1986) used observational techniques to study how health care workers manage risk of contagion in an AIDS medical research unit. Although observational methods appear not to have been used specifically to study older people and sex, they remain a promising option.

DATA COLLECTION INSTRUMENTS AND MEASURES

Because AIDS research is new and human sexuality is largely understudied, investigators have little previous scientific work on or established theoretical lines of inquiry from which to choose measures or develop promising research questions. Use of knowledgeable experts drawn from the population to be studied as well as ethnographic work can prove useful in mitigating this problem (Maxwell, Bashook, & Sandlow, 1986). For example, researchers at the Institute of Social Research at the University of Michigan collaborated with the Detroit area gay community in developing the research questions for a study of Chicago gay men (Emmons et al., 1986). The research team began by meeting with a focus group of gay males who were willing to discuss the risk of AIDS and how this threat affected their lives. Tapes of this gathering were content analyzed and the men's suggestions and reactions were used in formulating the study. Later, such informants provided a sounding board and validity check as the data were analyzed. The use of open-ended questions and semistructured interviews also provides a means to uncover information that might otherwise be neglected. Drawbacks are that such items are more expensive to gather; they also take longer and are more complicated to code.

Standardized Instruments

In contrast to building sex or AIDS instruments using insider expertise or open-ended questions, researchers who prefer ready-made scales and measures find few available. Those that have been developed have been divided into two classes by Conte (1983). One class uses Guttman scaling techniques to measure a cumulative pattern of sexual behavior, which assumes that subjects who "advance" to a particular measurement point will have experienced all preceding points. These scales tend to consist of about 10 to 20 items and cover a narrow range of behavior. Examples of Guttman-like scales for measuring sexual behavior include those by Brady and Levitt (1965), Bentler (1968a, b) and Zuckerman (1973). For an evaluation of these measures, see Conte (1983). Meanwhile, examination of the literature suggests that similar Guttman-like scales specific to AIDS have not been developed.

The second class of sexual measures uses questionnaires and inventories on a wider range of topics, information, and behavior in order to tap underlying dimensions. Conte (1983) reviews a number of these general measures (Derogatis & Melisaratos, 1979; Harbison et al., 1974; LoPiccolo & Steger, 1974; Thorne, 1966). In addition, examination of research on attitudes, knowledge, and behavior of the general public toward AIDS reveals a number of interview schedules that include at least one standard item on sexual behavior, and inventories designed for gay subjects tend to cover a wider range of sexually explicit topics and behavior (see, for example, Emmons et al., 1986; Joseph et al., 1987; Martin, 1987).

Measures of Sexual Knowledge, Attitudes, and Behaviors

Of the various instruments that are available, the Sexual Knowledge and Attitude Test (SKAT) is, perhaps, the most widely used. The test initially was developed for use with medical students, although it has been used repeatedly with other populations (Lief, Reed, & Ebert, 1972; Marcotte & Logan, 1977). Few of the items, however, have been specifically tailored for older persons. Only one question in the instrument refers to sexuality in old age, another to sex "beyond middle-age," and two to postmenopause sexuality. Experience also suggests that older people may be offended by some of the SKAT items. Brower and Tanner (1979) report that many people refused to participate in a study at a senior center where the SKAT was used.

Recognizing that the social and physiological properties of aging shape older people's sexual experience, White (1982) reports on the Aging Sexual Knowledge and Attitude Scale (ASKAS), which was developed for use with aged populations. The ASKAS consists of 61 items; 26 use a 6-point Likert scale to measure respondents' attitudes about older people and sex, and 35 request a true–false or "don't know" response to items tapping respondents' sexual knowledge. The knowledge questions query respondents about the capacity of older people to engage physically in or respond to sex under varying conditions. The attitude items ask respondents to judge the appropriateness of older people engaging in sex, particularly within the confines of a medical institution or nursing home. White reports that the scale shows high internal consistency when used with older people, their families, and nursing home staff (White, 1981; White & Catania, 1981). Several instruments assess the nature and extent of respondents' sexual problems. The Golombok Rust Inventory of Sexual Satisfaction (GRISS) is a 28-item questionnaire for assessing the existence and severity of sexual problems. The instrument consists of 12 subscales of: impotence, premature ejaculation, anorgasmia, vaginismus, noncommunication, infrequency, male and female avoidance, male and female nonsexuality, and male and female dissatisfaction. The GRISS and its subscales show good reliability and validity, although the instrument has not been tested specifically with older people. Other instruments or measures of sexual dysfunction have been developed by Derogatis and Melisaratos (1979), Harbison et al. (1974), LoPiccolo and Steger (1974), and Thorne (1966).

Measures of Attitudes toward Homosexuality

Scales that tap attitudes toward homosexuality are particularly relevant to current research on AIDS. Presumably the reputation of AIDS as a "gay disease" associated with a promiscuous and "deviant" life-style prevails among both the general public and medical professions (Conrad, 1986; Ostrow & Gayle, 1986), but a review of the literature suggests that these assumptions have not been scientifically tested. While many measures of homosexuality are restricted to attitudes of specific groups (such as college students and medical personnel) or focus more on homosexuality than on reactions to people who are homosexual (see Hudson & Ricketts, 1980), several instruments have been developed. Some of these differentiate between attitudes toward gay men versus gay women, a particularly critical distinction in AIDS research as gay men, and not gay women, are primarily the focus of fear and censure (cf. Gentry, 1986).

Among existing scales, Hudson and Ricketts (1980) developed a 25-item summated index of homophobia (IHP) that contains five items that differentiate by sex. Overall, the index is designed to measure the relationships between dread or discomfort in being around homosexuals and a set of biological, social, and economic characteristics found in the general public. Both positive and negative statements toward gay people and their interactions are included, and scoring ranges from those designated as "high-grade non-homophobics" to "low-grade non-homophobics." The authors report that the index has a coefficient alpha of .90 and a standard error of measurement (SEM) of 4.75. Various tests provide evidence that the index has high factoral, construct, and content validity. The appropriateness of the IHP for older adults is uncertain, however, as the authors tested the reliability and validity of the instrument primarily on college students in the social sciences.

Also in line with discerning sex differences, Herek (1984) developed the Attitudes Toward Lesbians (ATL) and Attitudes Toward Gay Men (ATG) 10-item scales that can be used separately or together. Scores on each scale range from 10 to 90, with higher scores indicating greater negativism. Herek (1987) reports the results of a recent study where internal consistency (alpha) coefficients for the scales were .86 (ATL) and .91 (ATG). Albrecht, Levy, & Sugrue (1987) report an alpha of .71 for the ATG when used in a recent public attitude study. These results support the value of using these scales.

Question Wording and Problems of Validity

A central problem in design and use of data collection instruments and the measures derived from them relates to the wording of questions and the meanings particular words convey both to respondent and investigator. In research on human sexuality, respondents' answers are likely to reflect highly charged attitudes toward sex that range from boasting to secrecy to denial (Siegel & Bauman, 1986; Wales, 1974). In AIDS research, the stigma of having the disease or being a member of a high-risk group may encourage people to be less than truthful. In part, these problems are countered by using interviewers with the social characteristics most likely to encourage respondent confidence and trust, or by careful structuring of the situation and setting in which data are collected. More generally, thoughtful wording of study instruments also encourages valid answers.

For example, gay respondents are more likely to answer honestly in AIDS research if they feel investigators accept their sexual choices. Such messages are communicable through the wording and phrases used in the investigation. One opportunity lies in the use of the term "gay" in preference to "homosexual." Although the latter term is not necessarily pejorative, Siegel and Bauman (1986) argue that gay is the preferable adjective for two reasons. First, it is a term that was adopted by people within that community to describe themselves, rather than one adopted by outsiders; second, it denotes a life-style that embodies many activities and values, not merely sexual behavior. The term "homosexual," however, may be more precise when describing actual behavior.

Overall, the general public does not have a clear notion of what is meant by the terms "homosexual," "bisexual," or "heterosexual." Both practice and identification with homosexuality and heterosexuality form a continuum, with men more likely to see themselves at the extreme end than women (Ellis, Burke, & Ames, 1987). When asked, people may not have a clear sense of where they belong relative to others. In other instances, the words themselves may be unfamiliar. This unfamiliarity is illustrated by a respondent in the pretest of the study by Albrecht, Levy, and Sugrue (1987). Having been asked if she considered herself "homosexual, heterosexual, or bisexual," the respondent paused before answering. Finally, after some thought, she informed the interviewer that she was bisexual. As the woman explained, reasoning told her that "bi" meant two, and she "always did it with her husband." Such confusion points to the need not only to clarify meanings of words, but also to train interviewers and coders in handling of problematic responses when they occur.

Another important caveat in the wording of instruments concerns terms related to the clinical aspects of AIDS. Many people in the general public and the professions are confused about the differences between having AIDS and being infected with the HIV virus. Researchers often introduce misconceptions about these disorders into their survey instruments. For example, one cannot "catch" or "transmit" AIDS, although this wording is common to many AIDS studies. Rather, people "catch" or become infected with the HIV virus; only later may they develop the associated set of symptoms and related diseases known as AIDS.

The misuse of clinical terms and phrases has important consequences for the validity of a study. For instance, a common knowledge item in many surveys asks respondents to indicate if they think people can "catch" or get AIDS through unsafe sex. In such instances, during analyses, it is impossible to evaluate whether or not answering "no" indicates little knowledge of the disease or a sophisticated understanding of the clinical fallacy built into this statement. Unfortunately, once the data are collected, it is too late to tease out these differences.

REFUSALS AND MISSING DATA

In addition to threats to validity raised during instrumentation, research findings on sensitive topics may be compromised when a large portion of a sample refuse to participate. Such refusals are particularly damaging when they reflect a trait being measured in the study or characteristics necessary for the sample to be representative. For example, people who prefer not to answer questions about sexuality may represent a conservative sexual viewpoint. Their self-exclusion from the study distorts or limits the generalizability of its findings.

A second threat to validity at the participatory level occurs when respondents systematically refuse to answer particular questions or sets of questions, so that missing values in the data are statistically correlated instead of being randomly distributed. This problem occurs in research on sex or AIDS when respondents refuse to answer two or more threatening questions for the same or similar reasons. Because attitudes about these subjects represent deeply held convictions and values, nonresponse on these topics is likely to follow a pattern. Given these concerns, what can be done to encourage prospective subjects to participate while discouraging item refusals?

Strategies for Encouraging Participation

As is true for research in general, people are more inclined to participate in a study if assured that their cooperation will be kept in confidence. This assurance is especially important with studies of gay men, as researchers often have poorly understood their fear of exposure (Cassens, 1985). Cooperation based on trust also is enhanced by having a sponsor and motive that respondents consider legitimate. For example, these factors are believed responsible for a research team's recent success in drawing a random probability sample of self-identified gay and bisexual male residents of the city and county of San Francisco, California (Bye, 1984). Media coverage concerning the danger of AIDS or describing the importance of the study also enhances cooperation (see Ginzburg et al., 1986). In general, when respondents perceive that the subject matter of the research is salient, their response rate is high (Senf, 1987).

Reduction of refusals also can be achieved through careful interviewer training, pretests, and pilot studies. The interviewers must have a clear statement of the purpose of the study that motivates the individuals to be interviewed, but does not bias the respondent. In preparation for the Albrecht, Levy, and Sugrue (1987) study, for example, the Survey Research Laboratory of the University of Illinois used a self-selection procedure in which seasoned interviewers chose to work on the AIDS study over other available options (Binson, Murphy, & Kerr, 1987). In addition, the Survey

Research Laboratory staff spent time during the training sessions helping interviewers to converse comfortably about both sex and AIDS so that they could transmit this feeling to respondents. This effort included practicing out loud sexually explicit words and phrases contained in the interview schedule. Training also included briefing sessions where interviewers were taught accurate information about AIDS and provided with the opportunity to ask questions about the disease and its transmission.

Study compliance also can be increased by building interviewer–respondent rapport. With older adults, for example, it may prove advantageous to use older interviewers; gay men are believed to prefer being interviewed by other gay men (Bye, 1984). Nonetheless, using interviewers of similar characteristics may not be as important as is commonly supposed. Darrow et al. (1986b) examined the effects of sex of the interviewer and place of interview on the responses of 145 gay men and 57 AIDS patients in four cities. The data were collected using five male and three female medical officers at sites of the respondents' choosing. After adjusting for geographic differences, sex of the interviewer and place of interview seemed to have little influence on the answers obtained. Moreover, in AIDS research as in research generally, over-rapport between interviewers and respondents can influence respondents to shape their answers to fit what they think the interviewers want to hear (Siegel & Bauman, 1986; see also Cannell & Kahn, 1968; Hyman et al., 1954).

Even when creative and detailed precautions are utilized to minimize refusal rates, some people, inevitably, will refuse to respond. When this occurs, an appropriate procedure is for interviewers to ask these potential subjects why they prefer not to participate and, wherever possible, collect demographic information. Analysis of these data, along with comparisons of the sample with population estimates, can help to control for response bias. Careful accounting also can be made of the refusal rate by time, day, week, language, and sex of the respondent, initial contacts, number of callbacks, and so forth to help the researchers calculate accurate refusal rates and to some extent determine the type and conditions of the refusals.

As in research generally (cf. Berk, 1983; Heckman, 1979), in AIDS research refusals should be analyzed as carefully as possible and reported in the presentation of research results.

Item Nonresponse

Item nonresponse is a second source of bias on the individual participatory level. Although considerable strides are being made to deal with this threat to validity, little work has been done on such sensitive issues as AIDS (Turner & Martin, 1983). Strategies to reduce item nonresponse entail (1) careful attention to the content and format of survey instruments, questionnaires, and interview schedules, as discussed above and (2) the use of statistical techniques and software once the data are collected.

In respect to the content and format of data collection instruments, sensitive questions can be psychologically sequenced so that they come deep in the interview after rapport has been established. Experience shows that sexual questions should precede demographic items that may suggest loss of anonymity, with income questions positioned last. For example, a preliminary item analysis of nonresponse patterns by Albrecht, Levy, and Sugrue (1987) suggests that people may be more reluctant to reveal information about their yearly earnings than their sex life.

Setting and timing of interviews also make a difference. Wherever possible, interviews should be performed when the respondent is in a familiar place like home or work, and when they do not have an audience. Presence of an audience has been found to inhibit respondents' willingness and comfort in answering questions about sex or AIDS (Binson, Murphy, & Kerr, 1987). Moreover, illness is of particular concern in studies of people with AIDS, although those who are sick vary in physical strength and functional ability. As the disease progresses, people with the disorder may find it increasingly difficult to participate in long interview sessions or to speak on the phone. Consequently, interviews may need to be conducted in short sessions or time periods where the person's energy is at its highest (Siegel & Bauman, 1986). Pretesting can help to determine if breaking the interview into segments affects the validity of the responses.

Studies of elderly populations present similar health-related concerns, although opinions about the seriousness of the problem differ. While most older persons are healthy, alert, and active, others have severe health problems. Perhaps these health differences explain conflicting reports among social scientists. Some researchers report that older people tire easily. Others find quite the opposite: older people display more stamina in relating their experiences than the interviewers who listen (Gibson & Aitkenhead, 1983; Rowles, 1978). Further health-related problems arise with the minority of older adults who have AIDS or other medical conditions (e.g., Alzheimer's disease or other dementias that affect the validity of response). Individuals incapable of giving reasonable responses are sometimes dropped from the study population or substituted for by a surrogate respondent, thereby raising new questions about accuracy of findings.

Once the data are collected, available statistical techniques are sometimes used to offset the biases created through item nonresponse. One procedure is to delete all cases with missing values from the analysis. This procedure, however, has serious drawbacks when used with sensitive data, since the number of item refusals is likely to be large and to be nonrandomly distributed. Little experience has so far been reported in research on AIDS and sexual behavior for other strategies (such as imputing missing values using dummy variables).

In sum, item nonresponse is an important issue in the study of sex or AIDS because the sensitivity of these topics poses serious questions of data collection, analysis, and reporting of findings.

SPECIAL RESEARCH DESIGNS

Many of the foregoing methodological problems persist even in the more sophisticated designs, such as case control or longitudinal studies, or cohort companions, which afford precision or depth to the interpretation of findings.

Case-Control Studies

Case-control studies have provided valuable information on specific risk factors for AIDS in a number of different populations, including gay men and ethnic and racial minorities at risk (Becker & Joseph, 1988). In a case-control design, individuals with a particular disease or condition are selected for comparison with a series of individuals in whom the condition is either present or absent. Such studies often are paired with clinical and laboratory trials. Relevant to AIDS research are Schlesselman's (1982) observations that case-control designs offer numerous advantages. He notes that they are well suited to rare diseases or those with extended latency; they require relatively few subjects, resources, or time to implement; they pose no risk to subjects; and they allow exploration of multiple causes of disease. On the downside, however, they rely on recall or records of past behavior that may be difficult to obtain or validate; control of extraneous variables may be incomplete; difficulties exist in selecting the appropriate control group; the method is relatively unfamiliar and difficult to explain to medical communities; and detailed study of mechanisms of transmission is rarely possible.

Longitudinal Studies

Longitudinal studies are particularly salient for studies of sexual behavior because sexual conduct is embedded in social relationships, attitudes, and life circumstances that change over time. Students of sex and AIDS who focus on change and persistence in attitudes, knowledge, and behavior of older adults potentially encounter the many rewards and problems inherent in longitudinal design (see Maddox & Campbell, 1985). For example, research on the incubation period for developing AIDS after infection with HIV may lend itself to longitudinal design (cf. Maltz & Brodsky, 1988).

Schlesselman (1982) observes that longitudinal analyses offer several advantages when used to study the spread of disease. He notes that, at least in principle, they permit development of a complete natural history of the disease; allow the identification of multiple potential effects of a given exposure; permit calculation of rates of disease for exposed and nonexposed individuals; and allow more stringent quality control over the measurement of study variables. On the negative side, to study rare diseases they require large pools of subjects; a long duration of follow-up is necessary; change in the treatment or the social context of the disease may make the study irrelevant before it is completed; it may not be possible to control extraneous variables completely; and it is rarely possible to study the mechanisms of transmission in detail.

Cohort Comparisons

Cohort comparisons of data from a series of longitudinal studies may be the ideal method for research on sex behavior and AIDS against which other, simpler designs can be compared. In studies of aging, one of the primary threats to the validity occurs when age and cohort effects are intertwined. This threat is likely to occur in studies of sexuality at each stage of the life course, because attitudes and practices toward sex have changed over the last decades, and the differing values, attitudes, and behaviors in cohorts starting life at different times may reflect these historical changes (Christenson & Gagnon, 1965). For example, the introduction of birth control pills in the 1960s was followed by a marked change in attitudes toward premarital sex for women (Arluke, Levin, & Suchwalko, 1984). Similarly, older gay men, unlike more recent cohorts of gays, often express deep dismay and rejection toward the "open sexual promiscuity" that followed the gay liberation movement of the 1970s before the AIDS crisis (Lee, 1978).

Because of perceived changes in sexual norms, attitudes, knowledge, and behavior in this era of AIDS, it is important to design longitudinal studies where baselines are established against which future intervention initiatives can be evaluated. Unless, these studies include more than one cohort and follow them through the critical stages of the life course, however, the findings will be limited to descriptions of aging, sex, and AIDS by members of one particular cohort in one particular historical time. As Riley (1985; Riley, Foner, & Waring, 1988) has shown, just as longitudinal studies can correct a "life-course fallacy" (of interpreting age differences to refer to the aging process), cohort comparisons can correct a "fallacy of cohort-centrism" (of assuming that all cohorts grow old in the same way).

ETHICAL CONSIDERATIONS

The problems of gaining participant cooperation for a study of either sex or AIDS point to the sensitive and often threatening nature of the topic. Issues arise over confidentiality, informed consent, and the nature of the research report.

Confidentiality

Practices related to sexuality are highly value-laden and disclosure of respondent's behavior may potentially create public censure and harm. Similarly, AIDS is a highly stigmatized disease that evokes fear and anxiety among both people at high risk and the general public (Conrad, 1986). Consequently, the ethical mandate that requires social scientists to maintain confidentiality about study findings is critically important when studying sex or AIDS. Yet the nature of AIDS as a sexually transmitted infectious disease creates special considerations and ethical dilemmas for investigators in maintaining confidentiality.

Because AIDS is an infectious disease, hospitals, physicians, and laboratories are required by law to report all newly identified cases to the Centers for Disease Control. Medical professionals who engage in AIDS research must consider the ethical and legal demands on both the physician and researcher. Moreover, the obligations of social scientists who rely on medical personnel as collaborators or for help with securing facilities or a sample are also unclear. A tricky legal and ethical dilemma occurs for all researchers when failure to disclose information places someone at risk for possible infection and, perhaps, death, which may occur in contact tracing or network analysis. In such instances, the investigator may be judged legally at fault if it can be demonstrated that filing a report would have resulted in someone avoiding infection or expedited recourse to medical treatment that could have prolonged life (Hermann, 1987). Yet violating a promise of research confidentiality can render the physician or researcher legally liable if it can be shown that that information harmed the person's interests (Hermann, 1987).

To date, a common strategy to handle this problem is to avoid gaining knowledge of AIDS wherever possible. For instance, surveys that ask respondents if they have been tested for the presence of the AIDS antibodies do not ask them to report the results of this test. Yet while avoiding possession of harmful information may sidestep legal and ethical problems, maintaining ignorance is not always possible. Thus ethics demand that researchers be realistic about the level of confidentiality that they can promise participants, particularly in research involving clinic populations. Legal concerns of the researcher in AIDS studies may include informing potential subjects of research limitations and securing legal counsel to ensure that the rights of the respondents, their social contacts, and the investigator are protected.

Informed Consent

Informed consent procedures ensure that subjects under scrutiny in sensitive areas understand any risks entailed in participating in a study. Informed consent consists of three requirements. First, potential subjects must receive full information about the study's risks, participation requirements, and the researcher's intended use of the data (Tanke & Tanke, 1982). This mandate often is difficult to meet in AIDS research because so little is known about the disease or its successful treatment. Also, with the rapid dissemination of new ideas and findings characteristic of AIDS research, investigators may find that their research interests and understanding of the disease undergo change as the study proceeds. This transformation is particularly common when using qualitative methods, where the direction and aims of a study are most likely to shift or to be clarified as the investigation develops (Roth, 1962).

The track record for fully informing subjects about what to expect in research of AIDS has not always been good. In the earliest days of AIDS research, the stigma and uncertainty surrounding the disease made it difficult to recruit sufficient numbers of subjects. As knowledge of the health consequences of having AIDS became better known, studies using clinical trials were besieged by applicants hoping to benefit from treatment (Levine, 1986). In some instances, people agreed to participate in a screening study in hope of personal gain, only to find that there was no follow-up counseling or treatment (Ebbesen, Melbye, & Beckmann, 1986).

A second requirement of informed consent is that subjects must not feel that they were coerced to participate in a study and withdrawal must be possible at any time and without costs. Honoring this rule is particularly critical in AIDS research where subjects have been recruited from clinic populations, so that potential subjects do not perceive that treatment is contingent on study participation. Such assurances may be more readily accepted if subjects are assured that their health care providers will not be told of their participation decision (Siegel & Bauman, 1986).

The third requirement of informed consent is that potential subjects must be mentally competent to make an informed decision. This issue is likely to emerge in studies of people coping with AIDS or of nursing home residents' attitudes toward sharing facilities with AIDS patients. In these instances, cognitive or emotional impairment can often impede the assimilation of information needed to make an informed judgment (Carnerie, 1987). Dementia, which affects many older people, is also a common degenerative stage among people who develop AIDS (Price et al., 1988). Analgesics or therapeutic interventions such as chemotherapy pose further barriers to gaining informed consent.

The legal guardian of a potential subject can give informed consent in cases where the person is mentally impaired. Such consent often is difficult to arrange, as families frequently may be reluctant to declare a loved one legally incompetent. Moreover, the use of a family member or guardian as proxy potentially interferes with the right of the person to confidentiality, a concern of particular salience in stigmatizing conditions like AIDS (Carnerie, 1987).

Even with optimal concern, however, no guarantees exist that all respondents will understand the information that is given. Early studies identified the issues here. For example, Dodd and Modd (1981) found that patients had little recall of information on drug use and side effects despite earlier having said they understood what they were told. Another study showed that although the quality of reasoning for elderly persons equaled that of younger patients, older persons did demonstrate significantly poorer comprehension of the information disclosed to them (Stanley et al., 1984).

Carnerie (1987) suggests several strategies for handling such problems. Subjects who have experienced a catastrophic illness can be given a period of time, perhaps several weeks, to deal with the crisis before being asked to participate in a study, although adoption of this measure impedes the schedule for data collection. Further, time permitting, the person can be given a copy of the completed but unsigned consent form to study overnight or longer. Over the course of the study, further opportunities may exist for information to be repeated and reinforced as new questions arise and people's conditions or perceptions change.

If blood tests are included as part of a social and behavioral project then other ethical considerations arise, in part those regarding protection of human subjects and those pertaining to testing for AIDS (see Carnerie, 1987).

Reporting Research Findings

A final ethical caveat pertains to how investigators report their findings. High mortality and morbidity associated with AIDS has led to great pressure for early release of research reports. The Assistant Secretary of Health and Human Services, for example, has urged all major journals to expedite review and publication of findings about AIDS and to allow prepublication announcements of findings (Stanley et al., 1986). In response, the *New England Journal of Medicine* announced it would suspend the "Inglefinger" rule that prohibits publication of findings already released to the public (Relman, 1985). The popular press and electronic media also have eagerly transmitted the news (Baker, 1986).

This market for AIDS and sex information has resulted in a proliferation of new studies, conflicting facts, and increased rivalry among researchers and health officials (Eisenberg, 1986). In the process, data and hypotheses have occasionally been reported without being adequately tested or controlled (Grodin, Kaminow, & Sassowen, 1986). Errors in the data or conclusions are common in any preliminary report. As a result, continual research updates are necessary to redefine, negate, or clarify earlier reports if the public and professional communities are not to become further confused and lose confidence altogether in any scientific guidelines for appropriate behavior.

BROADER IMPLICATIONS OF RESEARCH ON SEX AND AIDS

The study of sexual behavior and AIDS has extrinsic as well as intrinsic value. It can add to understanding of the life-course dynamics and the interactive social networks of sexually active older adults and persons with AIDS. It can provide a knowledge base for professional practice and public policy on AIDS. But in addition, it can feed back into broader questions of theory, method, and knowledge.

At the methodological frontiers, AIDS research already has made contributions to strategies for obtaining valid responses to sensitive questions. AIDS studies have compelled social scientists, epidemiologists, and physicians to collaborate on difficult and complex problems, an interaction that has resulted in diffusion and sophistication of research methods. Network research on AIDS can sharpen the techniques for measuring indirect influences in primary groups. Research in these areas has also emphasized the utility and importance of simultaneously employing different methods of data collection to cross-validate findings.

Studies of the sexual and AIDS-related behavior of older people can also add to understanding of social, cognitive, and behavioral theory. They force examination of the interrelationships among threats (such as AIDS), behavior, fear, and the quality of life. They examine the preservation and transmission of social and cultural values. The interdisciplinary nature of the work can also tighten the bond between biophysiological and social theories.

Investigations in this area, if carefully designed and analyzed, can provide results simultaneously on three topics: sexual attitudes and behaviors, older people over the life course, and AIDS. Such work is desirable because it has significant theoretical and practical implications.

Research in the fast-paced world of both AIDS and aging serves as a model for assessing the tradeoffs among speed of acquiring critical information, truth, and utility. In principle, speed, truth, and utility are all desirable. Yet, pragmatically, compromises must be made both for cost and for political reasons. Struggling with these issues intensifies understanding of the nature of applied social and medical research.

Furthermore, investigations of the sexual and AIDS-related behaviors of older people force confrontation with issues of ethics and values in both the process and the findings of research. The outcome should be a more incisive and humane understanding of what can properly be done in the interest of science.

Finally, where will this work take us as social scientists? Is this but a temporary phenomenon, or is there something inherently valuable in this research stream? Our belief is that we will profit enormously from this work, as long as studies are theoretically driven and carefully designed. We are seeking some missing pieces of the puzzle that will tell us much about human behavior in social networks across the life course.

REFERENCES

Albert, E. 1986. "Illness and Deviance: The Response of the Press to AIDS." Pp. 163–178 in *The Social Dimensions of AIDS: Method and Theory,* edited by D.A. Feldman and T.M. Johnson. New York: Praeger.

Albrecht, G.L., J.L. Levy, and N.M. Sugrue. 1987. "Evaluation Component of the City of Chicago's AIDS Risk Reduction/Prevention Program." Project funded 10/1/86–9/30/87 by Centers for Disease Control, U.S. Public Health Service.

Arluke, A., J. Levin, and J. Suchwalko. 1984. "Sexuality and Romance in Advice Books for the Elderly." *The Gerontologist* 24:415–418.

Baker, A.J. 1986 "The Portrayal of AIDS in the Media: An Analysis of Articles in the *New York Times.*" Pp. 179–194 in *The Social Dimensions of AIDS: Methods and Theory,* edited by D.A. Feldman and T.M. Johnson. New York: Praeger.

Becker, M.H., and J.G. Joseph. 1988. "AIDS and Behavioral Change to Reduce Risk." *American Journal of Public Health* 78:394–410.

Beeson, D., J.S. Zones, and J. Nye. 1986. *The Social Consequences of AIDS Antibody Testing: Coping with Stigma.* Paper presented at the 1986 Annual Meeting of the Society for the Study of Social Problems, New York.

Bentler, P.M. 1968a. "Heterosexual Behavior Assessment I. Males." *Behavioral Research Therapy* 6:21–25.

———. 1968b. "Heterosexual Behavior Assessment II. Females." *Behavioral Research Therapy* 6:27–30.

Bentler, P.M., and P.R. Abramson. 1981. "The Science of Sex Research: Some Methodological Considerations." *Archives of Sexual Behavior* 10:225–251.

Berk, R.A. 1983. "An Introduction to Sample Selection Bias In Sociological Data." *American Sociological Review* 48:386–398.

Binson, D., P.A. Murphy, and D. Kerr. 1987. *Threatening Questions for the Public in a Survey About AIDS.* Paper presented at the 1987 Annual Meeting of the American Association for Public Opinion Research.

Bloch, T., and I.D. Nebenzahl. 1983. "Respondent Bias In Mail Surveys." *Psychological Reports* 53:1227–1230.

Brady, J.P., and E.E. Levitt. 1965. "The Scalability of Sexual Experiences." *Psychological Record* 15:275–279.

Brambilla, D.J., and S.M. McKinlay. 1987. "A Comparison of Responses to Mailed Questionnaires and Telephone Interviews In a Mixed Mode Health Survey." *American Journal of Epidemiology* 126:962–971.

Brower, H., and L. Tanner. 1979. "A Study on Older Adults Attending a Program on Human Sexuality." *Nursing Research* 28:36–39.

Butler, R., and M. Lewis. 1976. *Sex After Sixty: A Guide for Men and Women in Their Later Years.* New York: Harper & Row.

Bye, L. 1984. *Designing An Effective AIDS Prevention Campaign Strategy for San Francisco: Results from the First Probability Sample of An Urban Gay Community.* San Francisco: The San Francisco AIDS Foundation.

———. 1985. *Designing An Effective AIDS Prevention Campaign Strategy for San Francisco: Results from a Second Probability Sample of An Urban Gay Community.* San Francisco: The San Francisco AIDS Foundation.

Callero, P.L., D.V. Baker, J. Carpenter, and J. Magarigal. 1986. "Fear of AIDS and its Effects on the Nation's Blood Supply." Pp. 227–232 in *The Social Dimensions of AIDS: Method and Theory,* edited by D.A. Feldman and T.M. Johnson. New York: Praeger.

Cannell, C.F., and R.L. Kahn. 1968. "Interviewing." In *The Handbook of Psychology,* Revised edition, Vol. 2, edited by G. Lindzey and E. Aronson. Reading, MA: Addison Wesley.

Carnerie, F. 1987. "Crisis and Informed Consent: Analysis of a Law-Medicine Malocclusion." *American Journal of Law and Medicine* 12:54–97.

Cassens, B.J. 1985. "Social Consequences of the Acquired Immunodeficiency Syndrome." *Annals of Internal Medicine* 103:768–771.

Christenson, C.V., and J.H. Gagnon. 1965. "Sexual Behavior In A Group of Older Women." *Journal of Gerontology* 20:351–356.

Comfort, A. 1976. *A Good Age.* New York: Crown.

Conrad, P. 1986. "Fear of AIDS." *Social Policy* 17(1):51–56.

Conte, H.R. 1983. "Development and Use of Self-Report Techniques for Assessing Sexual Functioning: A Review and Critique." *Archives of Sexual Behavior* 12:555–576.

Darrow, W.W., E.M. Gorman, and P. Glick. 1986a. "The Social Origin of AIDS: Social Change, Sexual Behavior, and Disease Trends." Pp. 95–107 in *The Social Dimension of AIDS: Methods and Theory,* edited by D.A. Feldman and T.M. Johnson. New York: Praeger.

Darrow, W.W., H.W. Jaffe, P.A. Thomas, H.W. Haverkos, M.F. Rogers, M.E. Guinan, D.M. Averbach, T.J. Spira, and J.W. Curran. 1986b. "Sex of Interviewer, Place of Interview, and Responses of Homosexual Men to Sensitive Questions." *Archives of Sexual Behavior* 15:79–88.

Derogatis, L.R., and N. Melisaratos. 1979. "The DSFI: A Multidimensional Measure of Sexual Functioning." *Journal of Sexual Marital Therapy* 5:244–281.

Dodd, M., and O. Modd. 1981. "Chemotherapy: Helping Patients To Know The Drugs They Are Receiving and Their Side Effects." *Cancer Nursing* 4:311–318.

Ebbesen, P., M. Melbye, and J. Beckmann. 1986. "Fear of AIDS." *Scandanavian Journal of Social Medicine* 14:113–118.

Eisenberg, L. 1986. "The Genesis of Fear: AIDS and the Public's Response to Science." *Law, Medicine, and Health Care* 14:243–249.

Elder, G.H., Jr. 1985. *Life Course Dynamics.* Ithaca, NY: Cornell University Press.

Ellis, L., D. Burke, and M.A. Ames. 1987. "Sexual Orientation as a Continuous Variable: A Comparison Between the Sexes." *Archives of Sexual Behavior* 16:523–529.

Emmons, C.A., J.G. Joseph, R.C. Kessler, C.B. Wortman, S.B. Montgomery, and D.G. Ostrow. 1986. "Psychosocial Predictors of Reported Behavior Changes in Homosexual Men at Risk for AIDS." *Health Education Quarterly* 13:331–345.

Gallup Report. 1986. "Methodology." Report No. 247:31.

Gentry, C.S. 1986. "Development of Scales Measuring Social Distance Toward Male and Female Homosexuals." *Journal of Homosexuality* 13:75–82.

George, L.K., and S.J. Weiler. 1981. "Sexuality in Middle and Late Life." *Archives of General Psychiatry* 38:919–923.

Gibson, D.M., and W. Aitkenhead 1983. "The Elderly Respondent: Experiences from a Large-Scale Survey of the Aged." *Research on Aging* 5:283–296.

Ginzburg, H.M., J. French, J. Jackson, P.I. Hartsock, M. MacDonald, and S.H. Weiss. 1986. "Health Education and Knowledge Assessment of HTLV-III Diseases among Intravenous Drug Users." *Health Education Quarterly* 13(4):373–382.

Grodin, M.A., P.W. Kaminow, and R. Sassowen. 1986. "Ethical Issues in AIDS Research." *Quarterly Review Bulletin* 12:347–352.

Groves, R.M., and R.L. Kahn. 1979. *Surveys by Telephone: A National Comparison with Personal Interviews.* New York: Academic Press.

Hagestad, G.O., and B.L. Neugarten. 1985. "Age and the Life Course." Pp. 35–61 in *Handbook of Aging and the Social Sciences,* edited by R.H. Binstock and E. Shanas. New York: Van Nostrand Reinhold.

Hagness, D.E. 1984. "Hear Today, Gone Tomorrow." *Modern Maturity* 27:122–125.

Harbison, J.J.M., P.J. Graham, J.T. Quinn, H. MacAllistor, and R. Woodward. 1974. "A Questionnaire Measure of Sexual Interest." *Archives of Sexual Behavior* 3:357–366.

Heckman, J.J. 1979. "Sample Selection Bias as a Specification Error." *Econometrica* 45:153–161.

Herek, G.M. 1984. "Attitudes Toward Lesbians and Gay Men: A Factor-Analytic Study." *Journal of Homosexuality* 10:39–51.

———. 1987. "Religious Orientation and Prejudice: A Comparison of Racial and Sexual Attitudes." *Personality and Social Psychology Bulletin* 13:34–44.

Hermann, D.H.J. 1987. "Liability Related to Diagnosis and Treatment of AIDS." *Law, Medicine, and Health Care* 15:36–45.

Herzog, A.R., and W.L. Rodgers. 1988. "Interviewing Older Adults: Mode Camparison Using Data From A Face-to-Face and Telephone Survey." *Public Opinion Quarterly* 54:84–99.

Hogan, D. 1980. "The Transition to Adulthood as a Career Contingency." *American Sociological Review* 45:261–276.

Hudson, W.W., and W.A. Ricketts. 1980. "A Strategy for the Measurement of Homophobia." *Journal of Homosexuality* 5:357–372.

Humphreys, L. 1970. *Tearoom Trade: Impersonal Sex in Public Places* (2nd ed., 1975). Chicago: Aldine.

Hyman, H., et al. 1954. *Interviewing in Social Research.* Chicago: University of Chicago Press.

Joseph, J.G., S.B. Montgomery, C.A. Emmons, R.C. Kessler, D.G. Ostrow, C.B. Wortman, K. O'Brien, M. Eller, and S. Eshelman. 1987. "Magnitude and

Determinants of Behavioral Risk Reduction: Longitudinal Analysis of a Cohort at Risk for AIDS." *Psychological Health* 1:73–96.

Kaplan, H.B., R.J. Johnson, C.A. Bailey, and W. Simon. 1987. "The Sociological Study of AIDS: A Critical Review of the Literature and Suggested Research Agenda." *Journal of Health and Social Behavior* 28:140–157.

Kortarba, J.A., and N.G. Lang. 1986. "Gay Lifestyle Change and AIDS: Preventive Health Care." Pp. 127–143 in *The Social Dimensions of AIDS: Methods and Theory,* edited by D.A. Feldman and T.M. Johnson. New York: Praeger.

Kovar, M., and J. Fitti. 1985. "A Linked Follow-Up Study of Older People." *Proceedings of the American Statistical Association* 179–184.

Lee, J.A. 1978. *Getting Sex.* Toronto: General.

———. 1987. "What Can Homosexual Aging Studies Contribute to Theories of Aging?" *Journal of Homosexuality* 13:43–71.

Levine, C. 1986. "Commentary on AIDS: An Ethical Challenge for Our Times." *ORB* August:273–277.

Lief, H.I., D.M. Reed, and R.K. Ebert. 1972. "Sexual Knowledge and Aptitude Test." The Committee on Human Sexuality (eds.). Chicago: American Medical Association.

Livingston, I.L. 1988. "Co-Factors, Host Susceptibility, and AIDS: An Argument For Stress." *Journal of the National Medical Association* 80:49–58.

LoPiccolo, J., and J. Steger. 1974. "The Sexual Interaction Inventory: A New Instrument for Assessment of Sexual Dysfunction." *Archives of Sexual Behavior* 3:585–595.

Maddox, G.L., and R.T. Campbell. 1985. "Scope, Concepts, and Methods in the Study of Aging." Pp. 3–31 in *Handbook of Aging and the Social Sciences,* edited by R.H. Binstock and E. Shanas. New York: Van Nostrand Reinhold.

Maltz, M.D., and M.D. Brodsky. 1988. "Developing AIDS After Infection with HIV: Estimating Its Likelihood and Incubation Period." In preparation.

Marcotte, D.B., and C. Logan. 1977. "Medical Sex Education: Allowing Attitude Alteration." *Archives of Sexual Behavior* 6:155–162.

Martin, J.L. 1986. "AIDS Risk Reduction Recommendations and Sexual Behavior Patterns Among Gay Men: A Multifactorial Categorical Approach to Assessing Change." *Health Education Quarterly* 13(4):347–358.

———. 1987. "The Impact of AIDS on Gay Male Sexual Behavior Patterns in New York City." *American Journal of Public Health* 77:578–581.

Masters, W.H., and V.E. Johnson. 1966. *Human Sexual Response.* Boston: Little, Brown.

———. 1970. *Human Sexual Inadequacy.* Boston: Little, Brown.

Maxwell, J.A., P.G. Bashook, and L.J. Sandlow. 1986. "Combining Ethnographic and Experimental Methods in Educational Evaluation." Pp. 121–143 in *Educational Evaluation: Ethnography in Theory, Practice, and Politics,* edited by David M. Featherman and Mary Anne Pitman. Beverly Hills: Sage.

McKusick, L., W. Hortsman, and T.J. Coates. 1985. "AIDS and Sexual Behavior Reported by Gay Men in San Francisco." *American Journal of Public Health* 75(5):493–496.

National Center for Health Statistics. 1987. *Evaluation of Item Nonresponse in the National Medical Care Utilization and Expenditure Survey.* Series A, Methodological Report No. 3.

National Gay and Lesbian Task Force. 1988. *Anti-Gay Violence, Victimization and Defamation In 1987.* Washington, D.C.:Author.

National Opinion Research Center. 1987. *Social and Behavioral Aspects of Health and Fertility-Related Behavior.* Technical Proposal #NICHD-DBS-97-13. Submitted to the National Institute of Child Health and Human Development.

Ostrow, D.G., and T.C. Gayle. 1986. "Psychosocial and Ethical Issues of AIDS Health Care Programs." *ORB* August:284–294.

Price, R.W., B. Brew, J. Sidtis, J. Rosenbaum, A.C. Scheck, and P. Cleary. 1988. "The Brain in AIDS: Central Nervous System HIV-I Infections and AIDS Dementia Complex." *Science* 239:586–591.

Reinharz, S., and G. Rowles. 1987. *Qualitative Gerontology.* New York: Springer Publishing Co.

Relman, A.S. 1985. "Introduction to AIDS: The Emerging Ethical Dilemmas." *A Hastings Center Report Special Supplement* August: 1–2.

Riley, M.W. 1985. "Age Strata in Social Systems." Pp. 369–411 in *Handbook on Aging and the Social Sciences,* edited by R.H. Binstock and E. Shanas. New York: Van Nostrand Reinhold.

Riley, M.W., A. Foner, and J. Waring. 1988. "A Sociology of Age." Pp. 243–290 in *Handbook of Sociology,* edited by N.J. Smelser and R. Burt. Berkeley, CA: Sage.

Roth, J. 1962. "Comments on Secret Observation." *Social Problems* 9:283–284.

Rowles, G.D. 1978. "Reflections on Experiential Fieldwork." Pp. 173–193 in *Humanistic Geography: Prospects and Problems,* edited by D. Ley and M. Samuels. Chicago: Marroufa Press.

Schlesselman, J.J. 1982. *Case-control Studies: Design, Conduct, and Analysis.* New York: Oxford University Press.

Senf, J.H. 1987. "The Option To Refuse: A Tool In Understanding Non-response in Mailed Surveys." *Public Opinion Quarterly* 11:775–781.

Siegel, K., and L.J. Bauman. 1986. "Methodological Issues in AIDS-Related Research." Pp. 15–39 in *The Social Dimensions of AIDS: Method and Theory,* edited by D.A. Feldman and T.M. Johnson. New York: Praeger.

Simkins, L., and A. Kushner. 1986. "Attitudes towards AIDS, Herpes II and Toxic Shock Syndrome: Two Years Later." *Psychological Reports* 59:883–893.

Stall, R., L. McKusick, J. Wiley, T.J. Coates, and D.G. Ostrow. 1986. "Alcohol and Drug Use during Sexual Activity and Compliance with Safe Sex Guidelines for AIDS: The AIDS Behavioral Research Project." *Health Education Quarterly* 13:359–371.

Stanley, B., M. Guido, M. Stanley, and D. Shortell. 1984. "The Elderly Patient and Informed Consent: Empirical Findings." *Journal of The American Medical Association* 252:1302–1306.

Starr, B.D. 1985. "Sexuality and Aging." Pp. 97–126 in *Annual Review of Gerontology and Geriatrics,* edited by C. Eisdorfer, M.P. Lawton, and G.L. Maddox. New York: Springer Publishing Co.

Starr, B.D., and M.B. Weiner. 1981. *Sex and Sexuality in the Mature Years.* New York: Stein and Day.

Tanke, E., and T.J. Tanke. 1982. "Regulation and Education: The Role of the Institutional Review Board in Social Science Research." Pp. 131–149 in *The Ethics of Social Research: Fieldwork, Regulation and Publication,* edited by J.E. Sieber. New York: Springer-Verlag.

Thornberry, O.T., and J.T. Massey. 1987. *Trends in U.S. Telephone Coverage across Time and Subgroups.* Presentation at the International Conference on Telephone Survey Methodology, Charlotte, N.C.

Thorne, F.C. 1966. "The Sex Inventory." *Journal of Clinical Psychology* 22:367–374.

Turner, C.F., and E. Martin, eds. 1983. *Surveying Subjective Phenomena*. New York: Russell Sage Foundation.

Van, J. 1988. "Norwegian Family Got AIDS in 1960's, Researchers Report." *Chicago Tribune,* June 21.

Wales, J.B. 1974. "Sexuality in Middle and Old Age: A Critical Review of the Literature." *Case Western Reserve University Journal of Sociology* 6:82–105.

Weg, R.B. 1983. "Introduction: Beyond Intercourse and Orgasm." Pp. 1–37 in *Sexuality in the Later Years,* edited by R. Weg. New York: Academic Press.

Welch, S. 1975. "Sampling by Referral in a Dispersed Population." *Public Opinion Quarterly* 41:74–79.

White, C.B. 1981. "Interest, Attitudes, Knowledge, and Sexual Behavior in the Institutionalized." *Archives of Sexual Behavior* 11:11–21.

———. 1982. "A Scale for the Assessment of Attitudes and Knowledge Regarding Sexuality in the Aged." *Archives of Sexual Behavior* 11:491–502.

White, C.B., and J. Catania. 1981. "Sexual Education for Aged People, People Who Work with the Aged, and Families of Aged People." *International Journal of Aging and Human Development* 15:121–138.

Wiebel, W. 1987. Research Proposal Submitted to the National Institute on Drug Abuse. Project funded for 9/30/87–8/31/90. SRCD (13) 1R18 DA 05285-01.

Williams, L.S. 1986. "AIDS Risk Reduction: A Community Health Education Intervention for Minority High Risk Group Members." *Health Education Quarterly* 13:407–421.

Wolchik, S.A., S.L. Braver, and K. Jensen. 1985. "Volunteer Bias in Erotica Research: Effects of Intrusiveness of Measure and Sexual Background." *Archives of Sexual Behavior* 14:93–107.

Zich, J., and L. Temoshok. 1986. "Applied Methodology: A Primer of Pitfalls and Opportunities in AIDS Research." Pp. 41–57 in *Dimensions of AIDS,* edited by D.A. Feldman and T.M. Johnson. New York: Praeger.

Zuckerman, M. 1973. "Scales for Sex Experience for Males and Females." *Journal of Consulting and Clinical Psychology* 41:27–29.

PART III

Care

CHAPTER 7

On the Relevance of Social Science Concepts and Perspectives

John B. McKinlay, Katherine Skinner,
John W. Riley, Jr., and Diane Zablotsky

> If men could learn from history, what lessons it might teach us! But passion and party blind our eyes, and the light which experience gives us is a lantern on the stern, which shines only on the waves behind us!
>
> Samuel Taylor Coleridge

It is impossible to overstate the magnitude of the impact of AIDS on individuals across their adult lives, and on their families and friends, the health care system, and the larger society in which they live. Yet the challenge of understanding the depth and dimensions of this impact on people of all ages has not been met. As an aid in meeting this challenge, which is the theme of this chapter, much earlier work in the social sciences links with work in the biomedical sciences to provide perspectives that are relevant for understanding the impact of AIDS. Thus research on AIDS need not start from scratch. And currently developing theories of health behaviors and health care in respect to AIDS can benefit—to borrow from Coleridge—by placing the lantern of social science experience on the bow, where it can shine on the waves ahead.

This chapter takes note of the benefit of selected concepts and perspectives from the social sciences for:

1. interpreting research findings
2. designing further research, and
3. using the accumulating knowledge as a basis for interventions.

The opening section of the chapter points to the historical parallelism between AIDS and other epidemics, emphasizing the point that biological knowledge is not a necessary prerequisite for effective social action and public health programs. The second section provides selected examples of sociological concepts and perspectives on AIDS patients, their attitudes and behaviors, and their social networks; and the third section provides further examples of their treatment and the formal and informal systems of care in which they are embedded. The chapter concludes with a conceptual model of the pathogenesis of AIDS viewed as an "illness career," together with an illustrative agenda of issues in need of research, and an indication of points already demanding social intervention.

Throughout the chapter, the implications of AIDS for persons in the middle and later years of life will be noted. Today, AIDS strikes primarily people under age 40 (nearly half of the new cases each year are aged 30–39—see the chapter in this volume by Stall, Catania, & Pollack). There are, however, at least three reasons for giving special attention to people in their middle and later years. First, already one fifth of the new cases of AIDS each year are in their forties, and another one tenth are 50 and over. Second, since the HIV virus may remain latent for many years before surfacing, the unknown numbers of people already infected are aging during the long period of incubation: those now in their forties will soon be in their fifties; and those now 50 and over will soon be 60 and over. (For further discussion of these points, see Chapter 1 in this volume; see also the chapter by Maddox and Maddox.) And third, it is clear that many older persons will be the givers, rather than the receivers, of care and support to AIDS patients who are young.

SOME LESSONS FROM HISTORY

Given the present state of knowledge and the national response to AIDS, the words from Coleridge at the beginning of this chapter are particularly apt, for the emerging response to AIDS is largely ahistorical. Yet there are significant implications for current public policy on AIDS to be gleaned from history.

When John Snow in the dead of night removed the handle of the Broad Street pump, he had as little understanding of the disease mechanisms of cholera as we have of AIDS today. Back in Victorian England he knew that, somehow, cholera was transmitted through water supplied by the Southwark and Vauxhall Companies. His community experiment (removing the pump) resulted in the dramatic reduction of cholera in nineteenth-century London (Hill, 1955; Snow, 1855). Specific knowledge of the biology of the disease and its waterborne pathways did not follow until many years later. A comparable situation existed with Budd's rejection in 1839 of the prevailing miasmatic origin of typhoid fever in favor of the view that it is "contagious and self propagating" (Budd, 1873). It was not until many years later (ca. 1880) that the typhoid fever bacillus was described.

The promise of community-based public health interventions, however, is certainly not limited to situations where basic pathophysiologic understanding is unavailable. It is now well understood that specific medical measures contributed relatively little to the decline in infectious disease mortality earlier this century (J. McKinlay & S. McKinlay, 1977) or to the more recent changes in the three major chronic diseases (J. McKinlay, S. McKinlay, & Beaglehole, 1988; forthcoming). Even for today's major chronic diseases—such as coronary heart disease, cancer and stroke (about which considerably more is known than is currently known about AIDS)—various types of public health interventions still appear to offer major promise. Confronted with the relative ineffectiveness of conventional one-on-one medical treatments for these chronic diseases, several federal agencies have opted for large-scale community programs in primary and secondary prevention (e.g., Rakowski, forthcoming). Input from historical experience as well as from broad social science knowledge has figured importantly in the design, implementation, and evaluation of these public health programs (the ongoing community demonstration projects in Minnesota, New England, and California emphasizing the primary prevention of CHD are notable examples).

In short, although the risk factors for these chronic diseases have been well documented, the underlying disease mechanisms have remained obscure. Nevertheless, community action has still been effectively initiated. Clearly, we can never know enough about the biological processes of disease, but we can know enough to proceed in the meantime with well-targeted social action programs.

A situation comparable to these historical precedents presents itself today with AIDS: while we presently lack full scientific knowledge of the pathophysiology of the disease, we have sufficient understanding of the modes of transmission (e.g., unprotected homosexual and heterosexual sexual activity, IV drug abuse, contaminated blood supply, perinatal conditions) to undertake community-based interventions targeted at known high-risk behaviors (see the chapter in this volume by Stall, Catania, & Pollack). Incomplete biological understanding (a situation that is changing rapidly) should be no obstacle to social programs for intervention.

Nevertheless, the essential ahistoricism of our national approach to AIDS is evident in the major preoccupation with the biomedical search for a cure or vaccine—something most researchers consider unlikely in the near future (cf. reports from the International AIDS Conference in Stockholm, 1988). As in the past, progress against this modern scourge will predictably result *not* from the immediate development of an effective and affordable "magic bullet," but from public health measures. In the first instance, progress will predictably result from protection of the blood supply, education in safe sex practices, the use of condoms, community health interventions directed at IV drug abusers, and the like. Yet it is evident that, as Coleridge put it, "passion and party blind our eyes" to historical experience and sound epidemiological knowledge with respect to AIDS. Commonsense strategies and even a willingness to experiment with innovative social approaches remain obstructed by political, professional, and religious interest groups (Shilts, 1987). This is evident in many aspects of the controversies over widespread reproductive education, the availability of needles for IV drug abusers, and accessibility to condoms for at-risk teens and adolescents.

Manifestly, then, AIDS is not only a medical problem, but also a social problem of pandemic dimensions. The onset and spread of the epidemic results from social behavior and produces social consequences. And it requires, at least at this stage of scientific knowledge development, social interventions. Even when the pathophysiology of AIDS becomes more completely understood (as is now the case for coronary heart disease and cancer, for example), public health interventions will most likely still continue to offer the most effective, cost-efficient, and socially acceptable approaches. Provided that they are appropriately informed by the social sciences, public health measures such as educational campaigns and community-based interventions with sound evaluation offer considerable promise, as history has demonstrated.

NOTES ON AIDS PATIENTS AND THEIR SIGNIFICANT OTHERS

Our primary concern in this chapter is less with the obvious relevance of social science to the etiology or the epidemiology of AIDS than with the consequences of the disease for older people. Our major focus is on two critical questions:

1. What can social science perspectives and research tell us about how this epidemic affects its sufferers and their significant others? and
2. What role can these perspectives and this research play in both the formal and informal systems of care?

Social scientists have long given thought to many diverse aspects of disease and disability in general, thought that now has potential relevance to AIDS. For example, their concerns have included: being "labeled" or diagnosed as sick and the adverse consequences; adopting the "sick role" and the changes this makes in the lives of patients and their family members; coping with these changes; fear of another's fear; ineffective communication and the failure to seek medical treatment; emotional support of the patient; and the many social and behavioral issues surrounding medical care (cf. Levine, 1962; Mechanic, 1962). This section will describe a few selected examples.

AIDS as a Label

To be officially diagnosed or—as in sociological parlance—"labeled" as having AIDS causes crisis and upheaval, not only in the lives of patients but also in the lives of their family of origin, their extended kin, and their friends. Early in the epidemic, official denial that AIDS was a threat to the health of the public at large was possible because the groups at risk were perceived as "different" from the rest of the population (Shilts, 1987), and most individuals could make personal use of such denial, averring that the AIDS risk "does not apply to me." However, it is now known that many who are neither gay/bisexual nor IV drug abusers will succumb to AIDS, and many may be infected with the virus and infectious to others, even when not officially diagnosed. Increasingly, distinctions are being made in clinical diagnoses that affect the "labeling" of the patient: there is not only the distinction between being HIV-seropositive and actually having AIDS; in addition, there are distinctions between the full-blown disease and the numerous serious opportunistic infections (which were formerly grouped together and labeled Aids-Related Complex, or ARC). As applied to patients, the distinctions among such labels have serious implications. They affect both the self-definitions of patients and the definitions ascribed to patients by others. And such definitions (or labels) affect an entire range of feelings, attitudes, and behaviors, from the patients' relationships with family and friends to the patients' experience with medical care. It is a well-established sociological principle that labels and self-definitions can become self-fulfilling prophecies.

The Meaning of Stigma

Closely related to labeling, and with similar significance for the understanding of AIDS, is the sociological concept of "stigma." Here the most insightful work appears in the writings of Erving Goffman (1963). Goffman began with an interest in "impression management," which denotes the efforts people make to create and sustain desired images about themselves and thus to control the conduct of others—especially their "responsive treatment"—by controlling the types of information they receive. Goffman's characteristic elaboration of the details of stigma and its management provide many subtle clues to be pursued in research and practice with respect to AIDS.

Goffman's extended work focuses specifically on the behavior of people with a stigma, or an "undesired differentness," of which he identifies three main types: (1) physical disfigurement; (2) aberrations of character and/or personality; and (3) social categorizations such as race, nationality, and religion. In short, "an individual who might have been received easily in ordinary social intercourse possesses a trait that can obtrude itself upon attention and turn those of us whom he meets away from him, breaking the claim that his other attributes have on us" (Goffman, 1963). Goffman argues that the type of impression management involved is largely a function of whether the stigma is invisible or visible, known about or not. If it is not immediately visible, the person is only discreditable and his/her primary interactional task is to manage any tension that results from the condition.

The subjective meanings for the stigmatized of their undesirable differentness are of central importance. For those with some permanent stigma, a viable self-identity must be sustained, while for those acquiring a stigmatized condition or entering a stigmatized state, a new self-identity must be created. The stigmatized are no longer what they had presumed themselves to be and must devote considerable attention to achieving what is vaguely termed "acceptance" by "normals." Goffman, among others, describes at some length the protective or defensive strategies that constitute the impression management repertoire of the stigmatized. Such tactics as "passing," "covering," and working out "lines" and "codes" of conduct help the undesirably different to cope with either discrediting or discreditable attributes and to protect them from mortifying situations (Davis, 1961).

It seems that the stigmatized are involved in a tortuous dilemma of self-contradiction. They are clearly denied any true acceptance in most social encounters, but they also—perhaps more importantly—act in such a way as to confirm the negative evaluation of their condition and thus remain stigmatized even in their own eyes. The paradox of such a situation is that, no matter how vast their repertoire of impression management strategies or how successfully these strategies are deployed to manage tension or information, the stigmatized remain wedded to the same standards of identity as do "normal" people—the very standards that disqualify them. Consequently, they are both other- and self-stigmatized.

One aspect of stigma that undoubtedly exerts an important influence on the utilization of health care (as summarized below) involves a person's self-identity. Denial of the existence of a stigmatized condition (for example, such AIDS-related conditions as skin blemishes) may be used to protect or postpone a change in one's self-conception and hence to postpone delay of recourse to medical treatment. Such denial is facilitated by the development of counterideologies, or self-rationalizations that the condition is unimportant, that others' evaluations are misinformed, or that the condition is only temporary and will pass with time (Davis, 1961; Garfinkel, 1967; Glaser &

Strauss, 1965). These self-rationalizations and the reluctance to alter behavior can be viewed as protective of those affected or their significant others.

These pioneering studies by Goffman and others on stigma, despite their direct focus on other types of "spoiled identity," are highly instructive as a guide toward understanding the reaction to AIDS. They not only point to hypotheses to be examined in future research on AIDS, but they can also inform the development of community intervention strategies aimed at ameliorating the consequences of the stigma attached to this disease.

Involvement of Significant Others

Once the diagnosis of AIDS is made, family and friends have to deal with the reactions of others. Here the extensive sociological research on "significant others" is relevant (see, for example, Kitsuse, 1964), but needs considerable adaptation to the fact of AIDS as a discrediting, if not a discreditable, condition (Goffman, 1963). Since various types of sexual contacts are widely recognized as transmission routes for AIDS infection, there may be lingering suspicions in the minds of family members as to the sexual orientation and perhaps promiscuity on the part of the infected person. Despite the substantial body of literature on stigma, there is little information on how stigmatizing conditions or states affecting younger family members also affect older people in the extended family. Because of the moral climate in which older people grew up, for them stigma may be especially devastating and disruptive. Except perhaps for studies of alcoholism, work to date on stigma and the societal reaction to deviance (labeling theory) tends to focus on the consequences of some condition or state for the individual directly involved (e.g., delabeling, deviant behavior, disavowal strategies), not on the family or network of significant others, including middle-aged and older family members and friends.

Understanding the functioning and response of AIDS patients' families and significant others is complicated because the at-risk groups are so diverse. Gay men and IV drug users are both stigmatized categories, but the family and social support structures of the two are very different. Blood transfusion recipients become members of stigmatized groups only after contracting the disease. Babies of infected mothers, whether or not they contract AIDS, may have no family who wants them or is physically or economically capable of caring for them. Even when such infants do not contract the disease, they may be unadoptable because of the stigma of the disease carried by the mother.

Fortunately, some pioneering sociological work on significant others is relevant to AIDS. For example, the study by Davis (1963) on sufferers from polio and their families provides a model for understanding the profound consequences for families of first discovering "officially" (through a diagnosis by a mandated medical labeler) that a member has AIDS. In the case of polio, Davis followed a small number of families through the transition from a state of relative security regarding their members through a state of severe disruption to ultimate acceptance. According to Davis, the American image of the "good life" is predicated upon the idea that calamity may befall others but will not touch one's immediate family. And it seems likely that with confirmation of the AIDS diagnosis, both the patient and the family (or significant others) experience a dramatic shift in self-image from a group more or less like other families, with a normal quota of satisfactions and troubles, to one that has been singled out for tragedy. While there are clearly differences and peculiarities in the ways particular families cope with such a crisis, there are enough similarities to permit a measure of understanding of an essential or modal crisis experience.

During the early stages of the epidemic, large proportions of the AIDS patients were reported to be young, gay or bisexual men, and the confirmation of the AIDS diagnosis was for some the first public affirmation of homosexuality. This open disclosure can be particularly troublesome for parents who, although suspecting it, may never have actually confronted the issue. While there are now fairly active committees for gay persons with AIDS, especially in larger cities, the effectiveness of particular counseling strategies is largely unknown. Nor are there means of ready access to supportive services for families or friends confronting the homosexuality of their loved ones.

Clearly, however, understanding of AIDS patients involves their significant others through every stage of the disease. Social science has contributed greatly to promoting and understanding the importance of significant others for the quality of life, but this work has yet to be applied specifically to the problems posed by AIDS.

NOTES ON TREATMENT OF AIDS PATIENTS

If the social science literature can provide a basis for understanding AIDS patients and their significant others, it can also contribute importantly to care systems in which these patients are embedded and the special experiences of AIDS patients in seeking both informal and formal support. (See also the chapter in this volume by Crystal.) This section focuses on care and treatment, although many of the same concepts and perspectives illustrated above are relevant here also.

Professional Care

The progressive deterioration in physical status associated with AIDS will, in most instances, eventually necessitate entry into the health care delivery system. With little previous initiation, the family is thrust into a world in which as much is left unsaid as is said, and in which the art of "hearing between the lines" comes disturbingly into its own (Davis, 1963). Medical professionals, socialized early in their careers to adhere to the biomedical model of disease, frequently have difficulty treating patients with a terminal disease for which there is no known cure. Earlier excitement over the discovery of the HIV virus has dissipated with the realization that the "magic bullet" may not soon be found. If AIDS follows the course of scientific development of most diseases, there will be many false starts and distracting promising reports (J. McKinlay, 1981).

Although physicians may not refuse to treat patients with AIDS, for many reasons there may be some understandable reluctance. Kelly, St. Lawrence, and Smith (1987) conducted a study in which a randomly selected sample of physicians in three large cities were asked to read one of four vignettes describing a patient. They then completed a set of objective attitude measures eliciting their reaction to the patients described in the vignette; these vignettes were identical except that the patient's illness was identified as either AIDS or leukemia, and the patient's sexual preference as either heterosexual or homosexual. Harsh attitude judgments were associated with the AIDS portrayals, as well as much less willingness to interact—even in routine conversation—when the patient's illness was identified as AIDS. Similarly, Lewis, Freeman, and Cory (1987) found that a majority of practicing physicians interviewed in a statewide survey "lack the AIDS-related knowledge and skills required to carry out their roles in dealing with AIDS."

Since increasing numbers of AIDS patients will be seeking medical attention, it will be important for health care professionals to develop programs that increase knowledge and counter the stigma and prejudicial attitudes associated with AIDS. Education is needed in this area because doctors and nurses trained in acute-care general hospitals may not be able to care for AIDS patients and their families in the community. The health care delivery system, which is documentably a frustrating hydra to patients with AIDS, appears ill-equipped to deal with the physical, psychological, economic, and social consequences of this devastating terminal illness. There is a disturbing parallel here between AIDS patients and seriously ill older people. A considerable literature exists on physicians' attitudes toward working with older patients—already a stigmatized category in the health care environment. Research indicates that many physicians spend comparatively less time and are less enthusiastic and aggressive with patients who are going to die from conditions over which the doctors have no control (cf. Haug & Ory, 1987).

Informal and Formal Care

Understanding of the interface between informal and formal caregiving in AIDS patients will afford optimum choices to the families involved. J. McKinlay and Tennstedt (1986) indicate that with respect to frail elders, there is no evidence to suggest the substitution of formal services for informal (e.g., family help); in fact, caregiving networks will ordinarily do "whatever is necessary" to keep dependent family members from being institutionalized. From the burgeoning social research on informal care, there is little indication that families withdraw their assistance in favor of utilization of formal services. While these findings from related areas are suggestive, it is not known if a similar situation exists for people with AIDS. Indeed, there may be substitution of formal services because the situation is different. The level of care may be higher because of the more acute nature of the disease, especially in its terminal stages, which necessitates more skilled care. Or formal services may be used more frequently for AIDS patients because of family fears of other social factors related to the stigma attached to AIDS patients (such as a public declaration of homosexuality), which may mitigate against family involvement in the care of an AIDS patient. Or formal services may be required when members of AIDS patients' support network are themselves sick or dying. But all of this remains speculative and certainly worthy of careful investigation.

Hospice care, however, may well prove to be the exception. Such care is the antithesis of hospital bureaucracy, for it brings both formal and informal components into one mode. The unit of care is the patient and his/her family, but the process of care is carried out under medically approved supervision. To be sure, while "relatively few physicians look to hospice programs when formulating treatment protocols for terminally ill patients" (Bulkin & Lukashok, 1988, p. 376), the AIDS epidemic seems likely to change the situation. Several social science research projects on the use of hospice care are reported to be under way.

Social Support

Highly relevant to the care of AIDS patients and their significant others as well is the concept of "social support," as elaborated by sociologists and other social scientists. It has been widely documented that the presence of social support (emotional support and instrumental aid as either perceived or actually provided) can reduce many of the negative consequences of stress, including symptom reporting, health-related restricted activity, and depression (cf. Elliott & Eisdorfer, 1982; McKinlay et al., 1988). Some studies exploring the mechanisms through which social support protects against illness have implicated specific changes in the immune system (e.g., Jemmot & Locke, 1984; Levy & Krueger, 1985).

In regard to AIDS patients, however, the influence of social support networks either on health or on quality of life has been given little research attention. Prior to advanced stages of illness, the AIDS diagnosis often means economic dependence since, as their physical condition deteriorates, AIDS patients are often unable—or may even not be allowed—to continue working. Sometimes in the case of two gay lovers, the sick partner may ask the other partner to leave. In other cases the lover may do the traditional caring, while all the time fearing contraction of the disease himself. At other times, and under different circumstances, the AIDS patient will return home or the mother will go to the sick adult "child." If there has not been successful meshing of family and friends, there is likely to be tension between the two sources of support. Research exploring the social support network of AIDS patients, particularly the interface between parents in their middle and late years and the typically young friends of AIDS patients, can have significant implications for management of the epidemic.

While investigating the existing support networks of AIDS patients, researchers are also challenged to find ways of supporting the members of social networks and investigating the relationships that exist among them. Investigations of caregivers for older people show that much can be done to assist their endeavors (e.g., through respite care, social support groups, information on formal care options); yet the degree to which caregivers for AIDS patients can benefit from the same kinds of assistance is not known.

The Role of the Family

Quite apart from AIDS, social research details the variety of conflicting obligations that can affect the family's ability to care for sick adult children (see, for example, the early work by Clausen & Yarrow, 1955; Sampson et al., 1962). One current conflict-producing trend is the large-scale entry of women into the work force; yet it is the women in the family who are typically the caretakers. While young and single women used to predominate in the work force, now the most common category of working women is middle-aged, married women (see, e.g., Bengtson & DeTerre, 1980). Despite such dramatic influences on the structure of the family, some adults with AIDS will go back to live (and die) with their family of origin. This will create a "renesting" phenomenon for aging parents who thought they had seen their children enter adulthood and achieve independent status (McKinlay et al., in press). The health impact of this nest refilling, particularly as it affects an aging mother who becomes the caregiver for an adult child with AIDS, is obviously not yet known. And for women in late middle age, the social and economic consequences of further delaying their reentry into the work force to care for an adult child with AIDS will have far-reaching social repercussions.

Still other social demands may be placed on the parent (usually the mother) of an AIDS victim. Since there are now many more people surviving to be old in our population, a middle-aged daughter frequently becomes a caregiver for her noninstitutionalized older parents as they age. When Elaine

Brody in 1981 called this generation the "women in the middle," she could not have foreseen the extreme demands placed upon a daughter providing not only informal care for elderly parents and perhaps spouse, but also the primary support for her own adult child with AIDS. Research on the impact of the physical, emotional, and financial demands placed upon these "women in the middle" is clearly indicated. Quite the same burden and its sociomedical consequences can also be applied to the younger women who will be expected to care for their elderly family members who have contracted the AIDS virus through blood transfusions or other transmission sources.

Care also imposes economic demands on families. Some of those required to care for their adult children with AIDS will be retired and living on fixed incomes. Research to see how people in their later years are coping with unforeseen and unplanned AIDS-related health care costs (estimated to exceed some $50,000 annually) is urgently needed. Clearly, whether or not particular AIDS patients, as their physical condition deteriorates, will come back to live with their families will depend partly on their socioeconomic situation, both current and prior to the illness. At the same time, their living arrangements will also depend upon the availability of significant others who are physically and emotionally able to provide terminal care. Again there are potentially relevant social science findings showing how social, economic, and behavioral factors are often more important than biophysical status in influencing a patient's living arrangements and interpersonal relationships (Kane & Kane, 1987). For example, one ongoing study (which refers to frail older people rather than AIDS patients) indicates that, contrary to popular belief, it is not the the sickest and most frail (by medical criteria) who are the heaviest utilizers of formal care: instead, several social factors (e.g., living arrangement and accessibility of network members) are at least as important in determining use of formal care (Tennstedt et al., 1988). This pattern may well pertain also to AIDS patients and their families. There is at least a sound *prima facie* basis for further research on this topic.

THE "ILLNESS CAREER:" A HEURISTIC MODEL FOR AIDS RESEARCH

The previous two sections of this chapter have illustrated some of the kinds of social science knowledge and theory that appear relevant for understanding the impact of AIDS on middle-aged and older patients, their families and significant others, and the health care systems in which they are embedded. However, such miscellaneous bits of knowledge and theory do not lend themselves readily for use in building a systematic research agenda. Nor do they readily lend themselves to the immediate task of identifying possible points of health care intervention—whether preventive, rehabilitative, or supportive.

In this final section, accordingly, we suggest how the available knowledge and theory might be organized within a single conceptual framework: the "illness career" model. Empirical findings and theoretical understandings are now available to unravel the various stages that are presumably encountered as an individual at risk becomes infected with the HIV virus, contracts the AIDS disease, and moves—almost invariably under today's conditions—toward death (see the earlier models by Kasl, 1986; Suchman, 1965a, b). Over the past several decades, the stages of transition from healthy personhood to patienthood have been studied more than any other phenomena in medical sociology (Mechanic, 1983; Zola, 1973), and the model has gone through various modifications, including special adaptations to the frail elderly and to incurable diseases, such as cancer (cf. M.W. Riley, 1983) and, in the present instance, AIDS. As traditionally used, the model has limitations: the stages are often overlapping and are not cognate with one another; and even more importantly, the relation to age needs further clarification. While the illness career is a process that occurs over time in human beings who are simultaneously aging, the career itself may be quite different if it begins in old age rather than in young adulthood. Despite such limitations of the model, it is useful for research on AIDS to delineate six typical stages of the illness career as these may be discerned in the findings of diverse social science studies and to identify at least one key AIDS-related research need at each stage.

At-Risk Behaviors

At this first stage the focus is on behaviors that increase the likelihood that an individual will contract the virus (e.g., hypertransfusion of hemophiliacs, IV drug abuse, unsafe or promiscuous homosexual or heterosexual activity). Primary prevention at this stage is designed to dissuade individuals from commencing at-risk behavior in the first place, while secondary prevention attempts to curtail already established at-risk behaviors (Baric, 1969).

To the extent that sexual transmission is involved, a crucial research need at this juncture is a systematic broad-based survey of sexual practices and attitudes, including use (or lack of use) of protective measures. At the time of writing, plans for such a survey are under way that will examine a cross-section of all adults in the United States. This survey is to include those in the postreproductive ages, who are least likely to be protected by contraceptive devices despite age-related changes in immune function and in vulnerability to infection through blood transfusion and heterosexual contact. The results of this massive study cannot come too soon, because current preventive measures are necessarily ad hoc, and they are based largely on surveys of the specialized enclaves in which the epidemic began, rather than on the great majority of the population as a whole. (See the chapter in this volume on methodological considerations by Levy & Albrecht.) As the Swedish Minister for Health proclaimed at the 1988 AIDS International Conference in Stockholm, "prevention is the only vaccine we have."

Symptom Recognition and Informal Care

At this second stage the focus is on the awareness that "something is wrong," which leads to lay consultation, lay referral, self-medication, and informal care by family or friends (Cobb, 1954, 1958; Freidson, 1960; Goldsen, Gerhardt, & Handly, 1963; Kutner & Gordon, 1961; Yarrow et al., 1955). Self-medication by AIDS patients has come to include use of various chemical substances imported from overseas, some of which were earlier proscribed by the Food and Drug Administration. Although the substitutability of self-care for conventional formal health care services is debatable (Fleming et al., 1984), some studies suggest that practices of self-medication and reliance on the "lay referral" system of relatives and friends may delay recourse to formal medical services or reduce the extent of their utilization (Miller, 1973; Stoekle, Zola, & Davidson, 1963; Sweet & Twaddle, 1969). The influence of cultural and social–psychological factors on the perception of illness symptoms has also received social science attention (Kleinman, Eisenberg, & Good, 1978; Leventhal & Leventhal, forthcoming; J. McKinlay & Dutton, 1974; Mechanic, 1983), but systematic studies of responses to the diverse symptoms of AIDS have yet to be conducted. Even less is known about older people's response to AIDS symptoms. For example, under what conditions are older people likely to recognize or label symptoms as associated with AIDS, and how do older people compare with younger people in this respect? Studies of care by family and significant others have been described in the preceding sections, but many of the implications for AIDS need investigation: for example, the coping and adaptive strategies of families of persons with AIDS, the consequences for older parents who must provide both economic and social support for an AIDS-afflicted younger relative, and the relationship between the AIDS patient's gay lover and his parents as providers of care.

Help-Seeking (Utilization) Behavior

The focus at this stage is on health and illness behavior (Mechanic, 1962) and on the search for formal (as distinct from informal) help. Here again AIDS research need not start from scratch. Zola (1964) has described the "triggers to action" that precipitate the utilization of formal services. Linsky's (1970) study of the influence of personal attributes in community reaction to mental illness provides insights and findings that should be explored with respect to

AIDS. Rushing (1971) also documented the influence of social class and other social characteristics (as distinct from medical considerations) that affect treatment. The significance of personal characteristics, as distinct from biomedical factors, in the treatment of AIDS patients assumes special importance in view of the fact that many of the afflicted are gay males, racial and ethnic minorities, and IV drug abusers. There is an impression that children with AIDS (both the vertically transmitted and hemophiliacs) are treated somewhat differently. The extensive literature on the behavioral model of health care utilization, as well as the economic barriers to seeking care, should also provide clues to needed AIDS research at this stage (Wan, 1988). What is needed here is research on how specific behaviors (including fear of stigmatization) enter into the process of making decisions about taking particular actions to seek formal help.

Encountering the Formal Health Care System

In the case of all illnesses, once formal services are utilized, explicit changes occur: a mandated "labeler" becomes involved, classification of clients occurs, an official record is created, and a prescribed regimen is begun. Numerous studies have documented the way in which, even in professional situations presumed to be neutral, nonmedical criteria (e.g., gender, age, social class, or race) influence clinical decision making (Haug & Ory, 1987). A seminal paper by Scheff (1964) in the area of mental illness suggests that diagnosis and treatment behaviors are influenced by the payoff for the providers as well as the patient. While the importance of errors in diagnosis (in either direction, Types I or II) are considered with reference to psychiatry, the utility of the expected value equation is evident with respect to the diagnosis and treatment of AIDS patients. Relevant to AIDS are studies of shame (Lazare, 1987) and stigma (Goffman, 1963) as they affect the medical encounter and subsequent utilization of care; such studies are to be found in the literature on the negotiations between the patient and the professional over diagnosis and treatment (Haug & Lavin, 1983; and see the discussion above). Much remains to be learned, however, about the special experiences and problems of AIDS patients in dealing with nursing homes, community-based facilities, and other components of the health care system (see the chapter in this volume by Crystal). And how do these experiences and problems vary by demographic characteristics of people with AIDS, and by routes of transmission of the virus? This is a research area of especially high priority.

Patienthood and Significant Others

At this fifth stage the focus is on the sick role and the patient's behavior subsequent to conferral of a label by the mandated professionals (Kasl &

Cobb, 1966; Mechanic & Volkart, 1961). In this role, the patient is expected to comply with the prescribed regimen and, when possible, to do his or her part in "getting better." To be found in this broad literature are studies of reactions to official diagnoses, coping behavior, the effects on family and friends, factors influencing compliance, and satisfaction with medical care. Also pertinent to this stage are studies of societal reactions to illness as a form of deviance (Parsons, 1951), social influences on therapeutic behavior (Roth, 1963), and responses to institutionalization (George & Maddox, 1988). Many of these studies may provide insights into AIDS-related behaviors. However, their value in this connection is limited insofar as a key element in the sick role is that it is conducive to "getting better." Even with frail elderly patients, in the absence of an incurable disease there is always opportunity for at least a modicum of improvement in health and functioning. Yet in the case of most AIDS patients, the outlook for recovery is poor; thus new research is urgently needed on how people with AIDS and their significant others cope with negative prognoses, how they operate to sustain optimal functioning, and how they manage the anticipated period of remaining lifetime. Unprecedented probes into the individual psyche and into the existential meaning of human relationships will have to be undertaken. The methodological and field work challenges of work in such sensitive areas are formidable.

Dying and Death

The most predictable stage of the illness career is death: everyone dies. Yet for the AIDS patient, as for others with a fatal disease, the predictability of death has a special salience.

On the topic of death and dying there has been a virtual explosion of social scientific research interest over the past three decades. Existing findings center around an array of topics, such as attitudes toward death, ethical issues in the use of life-sustaining technologies, adjustment to bereavement, suicide, funeral practices, and compression of the period of morbidity prior to death; and considerable attention has been paid also to the process of dying. (For reviews, see J.W. Riley, 1983; Marshall & Levy, forthcoming. For discussion of related issues, see the Chapter in this volume by Crystal.) Students of the topic are increasingly convinced that there is a "dying trajectory," which includes a "living-dying" interval and an emergent "awareness of finitude" prior to death that permits communication of basic meanings for both the dying person and his/her survivors. Many studies affirm that sociological death often precedes biological death, that people literally disengage from society into death, that the powerful "will to live" can be turned off so that the timing of one's own death can somehow be "managed."

For the AIDS patient who is dying, then, a considerable knowledge base is at hand, although many of the familiar issues are often intensified here. Thus further investigation is needed of adaptations of hospice care to the special circumstances of AIDS-related death. Studies are needed of the therapeutic potentials of communications among AIDS patients, significant others, caregivers, and counselors—including clergy and lawyers. Moreover, the deaths of persons with AIDS will exacerbate the ethical dilemmas concerning the allocation of scarce medical resources and the ability to choose life termination before the disease completes its painful course. In some instances such issues must be faced by family members, in other instances by nonrelatives, such as lovers.

A SUMMARY NOTE

The intent behind this discussion of the illness career model has been to suggest its heuristic value as applied to AIDS. Although far from exhaustive, the model brings together in a single approach many diverse pieces of knowledge and theory available from medical sociology and other social sciences, and it has organized these pieces in a form suitable for use in understanding significant aspects of AIDS and the associated social phenomena. As such, it is our hope that the model—and the more general discussions throughout this chapter—may serve three purposes in connection with AIDS in an aging society:

- to illustrate the importance of the social sciences, as they link closely with the biomedical sciences;
- to point to gaps in social and behavioral knowledge that should contribute to the research agenda;
- and, in the meantime, to highlight points at which public health interventions may already be feasible.

REFERENCES

Baric, L. 1969. "Recognition of the 'At Risk' Role: A Means to Influence Health Behavior." *International Journal of Health Education* 12:24–34.

Bengtson, V., and E. DeTerre. 1980. "Aging and Family Relation." *Marriage and Family Review* 3:51–76.

Budd, W. 1873. *Typhoid Fever: Its Nature, Mode of Spreading and Prevention.* Original Publication 1873. New York: American Public Health Association, 1931.

Bulkin, Wilma, and Herbert Lukashok. 1988. "Rx for Dying: The Case for Hospice." *The New England Journal of Medicine* 318:376–378.
Clausen, J., and M.R. Yarrow. 1955. "The Impact of Mental Illness on the Family." *Journal of Social Issues* 11 (entire issue).
Cobb, B. 1954. "Patient Responsible Delay of Treatment for Cancer." *Cancer* 7:920–926.
———. 1958. "Why Do People Detour to Quacks?" Pp. 283–287 in *Patients, Physicians, and Illness,* edited by E.G. Jaco. New York: Free Press.
Davis, Fred. 1961. "Deviance Disavowal: The Management of Strained Interaction by the Visibly Handicapped." *Social Problems* 9:120–132.
———. 1963. *Passage Through Crisis: Polio Victims and Their Families.* New York: The Bobbs-Merrill Co. Inc.
Elliott, Glen R., and Carl Eisdorfer (eds.). 1982. *Stress and Human Health: Analysis and Implications of Research.* New York: Springer Publishing Co.
Fleming, Gretchen V., Aida L. Giachello, Ronald M. Anderson, and Patricia Andrade. 1984. "Self-Care: Substitute, Supplement, or Stimulus for Formal Medical Care Services." *Medical Care* 21:950–966.
Freidson, E. 1960. "Client Control and Medical Practice." *American Journal of Sociology* 65:374–382.
Garfinkel, H. 1967. *Studies in Ethnomethodology.* Englewood Cliffs, NJ: Prentice-Hall.
George, Linda K., and George L. Maddox. 1988. "Social and Behavioral Aspects of Institutional Care." In *Aging and Health Care: Social Science and Policy Perspectives,* edited by Marcia Ory and Kathleen Bond. London: Tavistock.
Glaser, B.G., and A.L. Strauss. 1965. *Awareness of Dying.* Chicago: Aldine.
Goffman, Erving. 1959. *The Presentation of Self in Everyday Life.* Englewood Cliffs, NJ: Prentice-Hall.
———. 1963. *Stigma: Notes on the Management of Spoiled Identity.* Englewood Cliffs, NJ: Prentice-Hall.
Goldsen, R.K., P.K. Gerhardt, and V.H. Handly. 1963. "Patient Delay in Seeking Cancer Treatment: Behavioral Aspects." *Journal of Chronic Diseases* 16:427–436.
Haug, Marie R., and B. Lavin. 1983. *Consumerism in Medicine: Challenging Physician Authority.* Newbury Park, CA: Sage.
Haug, Marie, and Marcia Ory. 1987. "Issues in Elderly Patient–Provider Interactions." *Research on Aging* 9:3–44.
Hill, A.B. 1955. "Snow—An Appreciation." *Proceedings Royal Society of Medicine* 48:1008–1012.
Jemmot, John, and Stephen Locke. 1984. "Psychosocial Factors, Immunologic Mediation, and Human Susceptibility to Infectious Disease: How Much Do We Know?" *Psychological Bulletin* 95:78–108.
Kane, R., and R. Kane. 1987. *Long-Term Care: Principles, Programs, and Policies.* New York: Springer Publishing Co.
Kasl, Stanislav. 1986. "The Detection and Modification of Psychosocial and Behavioral Risk Factors." Pp. 359–391 in *Applications of Social Science to Clinical Medicine and Health Policy,* edited by Linda Aiken and David Mechanic. New Brunswick: Rutgers University Press.
Kasl, S.V., and S. Cobb. 1966. "Health Behavior, Illness Behavior, Sick Role Behavior." *Archives of Environmental Health* 12:246–266, 531–541.
Kelly, J.A., J.S. St. Lawrence, and S. Smith, Jr. 1987. "Stigmatization of AIDS Patients by Physicians." *American Journal of Public Health* 77:789–791.
Kitsuse, J. 1964. "Societal Relations to Deviant Behavior: Problems of Theory and Method." In *The Other Side,* edited by H. Becker. Glencoe, NY: Free Press.

Kleinman, A., L. Eisenberg, and B. Good. 1978. "Culture, Illness, and Care: Lessons from Anthropologic and Cross-Cultural Research." *Annals of Internal Medicine* 88:251–258.

Kutner, B., and G. Gordon, 1961. "Seeking Care for Cancer." *Journal of Health and Human Behavior* 2:171–178.

Lazare, A. 1987. "Shame and Humiliation in the Medical Encounter." *Archives of Internal Medicine* 147:1653–1658.

Leventhal, Howard, and Elaine Leventhal. forthcoming. "Vigilant Coping and Health Behavior." In *Aging, Health and Behavior,* edited by Marcia Ory and Ronald Abeles. Baltimore, MD: The Hopkins Press.

Levine, G.N. 1962. "Anxiety about Illness: Psychological and Social Bases." *Journal of Health and Human Behavior* 3:30–34.

Levy, Elinor, and Richard Krugeger. 1983. "Acquired Immune Deficiency Syndrome Is an Opportunistic Infection and Karposi's Sarcoma Results from Secondary Immune Stimulation." *Lancet* 52:680.

Lewis, C.E., H.E. Freeman, and C.R. Covy. 1987. "AIDS-Related Competence of California's Primary Care Physicians." *American Journal of Public Health* 77:795–800.

Linsky, A.S. 1970. "Who Shall Be Excluded: The Influence of Personal Attributes in Community Reaction to the Mentally Ill." *Social Psychiatry* 5:166–171.

Marshall, V.W., and J.A. Levy. forthcoming. "Aging and Dying." In the *Handbook of Aging and the Social Sciences,* 3rd edition, edited by R.H. Binstock & L.K. George. New York: Academic Press.

McKinlay, J. 1981. "From 'Promising Report' to 'Standard Procedure': Seven Stages in the Career of Medical Innovation." *Milbank Memorial Fund Quarterly* 59:374–411.

McKinlay, J., and D. Dutton. 1974. "Social-Psychological Aspects of Consumer Use." In *Consumer Incentives for Health Care,* edited by S.J. Mushkin. New York: Prodist.

McKinlay, John, and Sonja McKinlay. 1977. "The Questionable Effect of Medical Measures on the Decline of Mortality in the United States in the Twentieth Century." *Milbank Memorial Fund Quarterly/Health and Society* 55:405–428.

McKinlay, John, Sonja McKinlay, and Robert Beaglehole. 1988. "Trends in Death and Disease and the Contribution of Medical Measures." In *Handbook of Medical Sociology,* edited by H.E. Freeman and S. Levine. NJ: Prentice-Hall.

———. 1989. "A Review of the Evidence Concerning the Impact of Medical Measures on Recent Mortality and Morbidity in the United States." *International Journal of Health Services* 19:181–200.

McKinlay, John, and Sharon Tennstedt. 1986. "Social Networks and the Care of Frail Elders." NIH/National Institute on Aging Grant No. AGO3869.

McKinlay, S.M., R.S. Triant, D.J. Brambilla, and M. Ferdock. In press. "The Relative Contributions of Work and Three Nurturing Roles to the Health of Middle Aged Women. The Experience of the Massachusetts Women's Health Study." In *Gender, Health and Longevity: Multidisciplinary Perspectives,* edited by M.G. Ory and H.R. Warner. New York: Springer Press.

Mechanic, D. 1962. "The Concept of Illness Behavior." *Journal of Chronic Diseases* 15:189–194.

Mechanic, D. (ed.). 1983. *Handbook of Health, Health Care and the Health Professions.* New York: The Free Press.

Mechanic, D., and E.H. Volkart. 1961. "Stress, Illness Behavior and the Sick Role." *American Sociological Review* 26:51–58.

Miller, M.H. 1973. "Seeking Advice for Cancer Symptoms." *American Journal of Public Health* 63:955–961.

Parsons, Talcott. 1951. *The Social System.* Glencoe, IL: The Free Press.
Rakowski, William. forthcoming. "Concepts and Issues for Disease Prevention Research and Community Interventions with Older Adults." In *Aging, Health, and Behavior,* edited by Marcia Ory and Ronald Abeles. Baltimore, MD: The Hopkins Press.
Riley, John W. Jr. 1983. "Dying and the Meanings of Death: Sociological Inquiries." *Annual Review of Sociology* 9:191–216.
Riley, Matilda White. 1983. "Cancer and the Life Course." Pp. 25–32 in *Perspectives on Prevention and Treatment of Cancer in the Elderly,* edited by Rosemary Yancik et al. New York: Raven Press.
Roth, J.A. 1963. *Timetables.* Indianapolis: Bobbs-Merrill.
Rushing, W.A. 1971. "Individual Resources, Societal Reaction, and Hospital Commitment." *American Journal of Sociology* 77:511–526.
Sampson, H. et al., 1962. "Family Process and Becoming a Mental Patient." *American Journal of Sociology* 68:88–96.
Scheff, T.J. 1964. "Preferred Errors in Diagnosis." *Medical Care* 2:166–172.
Shilts, Randy. 1987. *And the Band Played On.* New York: St. Martin's Press.
Snow, J. 1855. *On the Mode of Transmission of Cholera,* 2nd edition. London: Churchill, 1855 (reprinted New York: Commonwealth Fund, 1856); reprinted New York: Hayfner, 1965.
Stoekle, J.D., I.K. Zola, and G.E. Davidson. 1963. "On Going to See the Doctor: The Contributions of the Patient to the Decision to Seek Medical Aid." *Journal of Chronic Diseases* 16:975–989.
Suchman, E.A. 1965a. "Social Patterns of Illness and Medical Care." *Journal of Health and Human Behavior* 6:2–16.
———. 1965b. "Stages of Illness and Medical Care." *Journal of Health and Human Behavior* 6:114–128.
Sweet, R.H., and A.C. Twaddle. 1969. "An Exploration of Delay in Hospitalization." *Inquiry* 6:35–41.
Tennstedt, S.L., J.B. McKinlay, L.M. Sullivan, and R.B. D'Agostino. "How Important Is Functional Status as a Predictor of Care for Older People?" Unpublished MS.
Wan, Thomas. 1988. "The Behavioral Model of Health Care Utilization by Older People." In *Aging and Health Care: Social Science and Policy Perspectives,* edited by Marcia Ory and Kathleen Bond. London: Tavistock.
Yarrow, M.R., C.A. Schwartz, H.S. Levy, and L.C. Deasy. 1955. "The Psychological Meaning of Illness in the Family." *Journal of Social Issues* 11:12–24.
Zola, I.K. 1964. "Illness Behavior of the Working Class: Implications and Recommendations." Pp. 350–361 in *Blue Collar World,* edited by A.B. Shostak and W. Gomberg. Englewood Cliffs, NJ: Prentice-Hall.
———. 1973. "Pathways to the Doctor: From Person to Patient." *Journal of Social Issues* 11:12–24.

CHAPTER 8

Persons with AIDS and Older People: Common Long-Term Care Concerns

Stephen Crystal

Research on the impact of the AIDS epidemic on the health care system, constituting a very small subset of all AIDS research, has concentrated mainly on medical care per se and particularly on its costs. However, AIDS has major implications for the long-term care system and other non-acute health care and related services. AIDS—or, more broadly, HIV infection—involves chronic as well as acute illness and is associated with a wide range of functional disabilities that include neurological and cognitive impairment (Grant et al., 1987), massive fatigue and weakness (Crystal & Jackson, 1988b), mobility limitations, and other symptoms affecting the ability to perform activities of daily living (see also National Academy of Sciences, 1986). Thus, the predictably increasing number of persons with AIDS (PWA), as well as an important and underattended-to number of persons with associated opportunistic infections (previously designated as AIDS-Related Complex, or ARC), are likely to require long-term care services (Crystal & Jackson, 1988a). This new group of clients must share the long-term care system with frail and impaired older adults and faces many of the same problems in securing appropriate care from that system. Thus this new demand on long-term care brings renewed attention and urgency to the entire range of chronic illnesses and to unresolved policy issues affecting the long-term care system as a whole, including problems of supply, quality, organization, continuity, and coordination of care; linkage between acute and long-term care; case management; and the appropriate roles of in-home and institutional care.

This chapter examines these persistent problems of the long-term care system as they affect both populations: those with AIDS and that minority of older people afflicted with chronic illness or disability. To be sure, there is an overlap between these populations (some 10% of new AIDS cases each year are aged 50 and over; see the chapter in this volume by Stall, Catania, & Pollack). But the focus here is on the similarities and differences between the two groups with respect to the organization, delivery, and outcome of long-term care. Also emphasized is the interplay between the two: as PWA utilize models of long-term care established originally for older people, the new and innovative models of care being developed in response to the AIDS epidemic can, in turn, inform improved long-term care options available to older people. Throughout the several sections of this chapter, the challenge is to enhance the knowledge base for providing adequate and cost-effective care to chronically ill persons without unnecessarily impairing quality of life; toward this effort, many of the same health services research and programmatic questions must be addressed for both PWA and older people.

NATURE AND EXTENT OF LONG-TERM CARE FOR PERSONS WITH AIDS (PWA)

The AIDS epidemic, whatever its future course (see discussions in the chapters in this volume by Manton & Singer and by Stall, Catania, & Pollack), is already having dramatic effects on those who work in the long-term care system, those who are concerned with its financing, and those (mainly older people) who must increasingly share that system with PWA. These impacts have received far less attention than impacts on the acute-care hospital system. However, long-term care supply shortages severely affect and are affected by the new demands associated with AIDS. While hospital bed supply problems have been significant in certain localities, preexisting excess capacity tended at least in the epidemic's early years to ease the strain on the hospital system. In long-term care, by contrast, little unused residential capacity preexisted.

Few data are as yet available on the sources and costs of long-term care for persons with HIV infection or the effects of supportive services on acute-care utilization or other outcomes. Much research needs to be done. Claims that particular approaches to supportive care (such as the "San Francisco model" —Silverman, 1987) create large savings in acute-care costs must be carefully evaluated in this context as elsewhere in long-term care; differences among cities or states in hospitalization patterns may have as much to do with the demographics of the PWA population as with care models. Comprehensive surveys of patient health and social services needs and utilization are required to provide basic data on utilization patterns and costs of supportive services for PWA.

In one study the figure of 13% of total health care costs was estimated to account for hospice, nursing home, and home care, and other long-term care costs of PWA (Hay, Osmond, & Jacobson, 1988, based on California data from Kizer, Rodriguez, & McHolland, 1987). Although this is higher than some other estimates, it may underestimate the actual burden for several reasons. As with long-term care of the elderly, much of the care burden does not appear in health expenditure statistics, because it is unreimbursed by private or public insurance or because it is provided by family members, lovers, and volunteers. Privately paid care and even in-kind care impose costs that are no less real for being harder to measure; volunteer resources may become exhausted as the number of ill persons increases, thus requiring an increased role for formal long-term care. Further, estimates of current and future needs based on the number or reported AIDS cases underrepresent the real health services needs. Persons with the opportunistic infections associated with AIDS, as well as AIDS patients themselves, may require long-term and other health care services which can increase current health care costs dramatically (Bloom & Carliner, 1988). Despite the "less severe" staging of their disease in purely clinical terms, persons diagnosed not with AIDS per se but with associated opportunistic infections suffer greatly from debilitating fatigue and other impairing symptoms and also report difficulty in performing everyday household tasks (Crystal & Jackson, 1988a). We refer for simplicity to the needs of PWA throughout this chapter, but it should be understood that the care burden includes and substantially exceeds that imposed by persons with full-blown AIDS.

PWA AND OLDER PEOPLE: COMPETITION FOR SCARCE RESOURCES?

Will frail older persons and PWA compete for long-term care resources in the future? For some while, little direct competition may occur, given current differences in the pattern of services utilized and, in particular, the limited use thus far of nursing homes by PWA. However, such competition is at least a potential concern, since the AIDS epidemic heralds a new source of demand in a situation where supply of long-term care and the dollars available for it are severely constrained. Existing research on social factors affecting both supply and demand provides a basis for understanding the potential for competition.

The pattern of holding supply of long-term care below demand through a variety of regulatory and financing policies, particularly at the state level, has been well documented, producing what one analyst has called a "state of excess demand in equilibrium" (Scanlon, 1980). Since the mid-1970s, growth in institutional long-term care supply in particular has been limited more sharply than was the case in the 1960s and early 1970s by such policies as certificate-of-need and reimbursement limitations, which exacerbate the imbalance. By 1980, certificate-of-need laws constraining nursing home expansion had been enacted in all but three states (Feder & Scanlon, 1980), and in the mid-1980s several states went further by initiating or extending freezes on the building of new beds (U.S. Senate Special Committee on Aging, 1986). Currently, regulatory authorities are faced with escalating demands for long-term care by older people. They also confront cost increases in other areas of the Medicaid budget; they are under pressure to improve quality deficiencies by requiring and financing enhanced staffing patterns; and they are experiencing the effects of labor shortages in many areas of the country that push up the wages of the long-term care work force. These conditions are continuing by and large to hold the line on supply of long-term care. For example, the vacancy rate in nursing homes (especially as contrasted with that in hospitals) is very low, and long waits for placement are not uncommon. This makes it difficult to reprogram facilities, or wings of facilities, to serve the PWA population.

Findings from the National Nursing Home Survey confirm the pattern of flattening of long-term care supply growth (Hing, 1987; Straham, 1987). The proportion of older people in nursing homes has remained roughly constant, but this apparent flat trend masks a real decline in supply relative to demand because of social trends reducing the availability of informal help. These trends include the continued movement of married women in their middle years into the work force, so that the likelihood of a caretaker being available to provide extensive personal care of an impaired elderly person is reduced. Recent increases in the proportion of women with even very young children who are continuing paid employment suggest that this process is continuing and will place even more significant constraints on the availability of informal help to elderly parents—or adult children with AIDS—in coming years. Also contributing is the continued trend to independent living on the part of the older person, so that a co-resident family member (the most prevalent source of personal care help) is less likely to be available (Crystal, 1984). Additionally, the more rapid growth of the oldest age categories within the elderly population—those aged 85 and older—contributes to the growth of long-term care demand at a rate greater than the overall growth of the 65+ population.

Thus, the long-term care environment into which the new demand for the care of PWA is introduced is characterized by a chronic and probably increasing excess of demand over supply. Despite some significant developments in in-home care, the primary source of formal long-term care for older people has continued to be the nursing home, and it is in that sector that the effects of supply limitation have been particularly visible. Tight supply is one of several factors explaining why nursing homes have not yet become a major factor in the provision of long-term care to PWA, though by no means the whole explanation. Hospital placement pressures and other factors could possibly change this pattern over time as the AIDS caseload grows, along with efforts now under way to make nursing home or other institutional long-term care beds available for PWA.

There are indications that spillover demand from the elderly population who cannot gain access to nursing homes is being seen in the home care sector. Some of the new need for care of PWA is also being met in this way. However, the work force for home care is finite, and in some geographical areas supply of workers has become a critical problem, particularly where unemployment is low. Thus, while in-home care is more "expandable" than nursing home supply, in this sector too there are real though less rigid capacity limits. The role of in-home versus institutional provision of long-term care services for PWA is an issue with significant implications for other long-term care consumers.

MODELS OF LONG-TERM CARE: SOME CURRENT PROBLEMS

In AIDS care, several new models are being tested or proposed, most of which are extensions or modifications of efforts to reorganize long-term care services for the elderly. Thus, as new models are developed and tested for PWA, providers and funders are frequently forced to address anew the familiar problems of case management and coordination of multiple services in long-term care and to develop new organizational solutions to some of these problems. The long-term care system for older persons has long been plagued by a lack of coordination with acute care, by absence of effective case management capability, and by the difficulty in flexibly modifying and adapting service delivery configurations to changes over time in patient conditions and needs. These deficiencies, problematic for the elderly population, may be even more critical in the care of PWA, given the rapid changes in their medical conditions and needs for care.

Nursing homes have not yet been widely utilized in the care of PWA, notwithstanding the often very substantial needs of this population both for personal care and technical nursing care. In New Jersey, for example, it was reported early in 1988 that not a single AIDS patient resided in a nursing home (Caplan, forthcoming). Efforts at placement in nursing homes have often met with resistance, either on the part of those facilities' elderly patients and their relatives or on the part of the facilities' managers. In New Jersey, plans were to have gone into effect in 1988 for use of half of one nursing home's 240 beds for PWA. However, the plans were suspended in the wake of protests from what was described in the press as an "angry mob" led by the town's mayor (*New Brunswick Home News*, 1988). (Later, some AIDS patients were placed in the facility.) In this instance, fear of contagion appeared to be a principal reason for resistance by some elderly patients. Nursing home operators have sometimes felt that they would lose their ability to recruit elderly patients if they admitted PWA.

In-home care, by contrast, has been widely utilized to minimize unnecessary hospitalization. In-home care, however, requires that the patient have easy access to outpatient medical and social services, often including home visits of professional personnel. Models for coordinated medical and supportive care are being widely tested.

In-Home and Community-Based Services

While detailed data on in-home care provision to PWA are scarce, such care in some cases is made available in more intensive service patterns than is the case for the elderly. This is undoubtedly a response in part to the simple unavailability of nursing home beds, to what may be a lack of acceptability of nursing homes to PWA themselves, and perhaps to the limited life expectancy of PWA. On the basis of their prognosis, most PWA can qualify for hospice benefits, though sometimes with a bit of stretching of the usual eligibility criteria.

Experiments currently under way in the innovative configuration, financing, and delivery of community-based long-term care services for PWA have clear relevance for elderly consumers and potential consumers of long-term care. Particularly significant are home and community-based waivers in Medicaid programs. As of mid-1988, programs had been approved in New Jersey, New Mexico, Ohio, and Hawaii, with the New Jersey program the largest. As one example, the New Jersey program, the AIDS Community Care Alternatives Program (ACCAP), was initiated in March of 1987. ACCAP permits addition of a number of services not normally provided under Medicaid, including case management, private duty nursing, medical day care, and personal care assistant services. Expenditures per case were capped at the cost of institutional care that would otherwise be required—the comparison generally applied being to hospital rather than to nursing home costs. This program represents a major long-term care policy initiative: 265 individuals had been served by the spring of 1988, with the waiver authorizing service to up to 1000 individuals at a time by 1989. By mid-1988, several additional states had AIDS-specific waiver requests pending, and others were using waivers originally developed primarily for older people in order to provide special services to PWA (Knickman, Benjamin, & Dunham, 1988).

These home- and community-based waiver programs tend to emphasize the provision of more extensive in-home services, such as private duty nursing and personal care, than is typically available through the regular Medicaid program. Such programs play a crucial role in maintaining patients in the community and avoiding unnecessary hospitalization. In doing so they also provide potentially useful lessons for home care for the elderly.

Several other model programs are complementing the home and community care waiver programs, such as the demonstration programs for the care of PWA funded by the Robert Wood Johnson Foundation (nine such programs were funded by mid-1988 in 11 cities) and the programs supported by the federal Health Resources and Services Administration (10 programs by mid-1988). While some of these programs have been hospital-based, such as the Robert Wood Johnson Foundation-funded projects in Newark and Jersey City, others have emphasized a community base (Knickman, Benjamin, & Dunham, 1988).

Little evaluation has yet been done on these programs, so many questions remain thus far unanswered. Community-based as well as hospital-based programs each have their own set of advantages and disadvantages. Hospital-based programs are likely to encounter discontinuities in care, particularly where more than one medical provider is used, and they often fail to focus on the home setting where the client spends, or should spend, most of his/her time. Community-based programs, when based on experience with case management programs for older people, may function well in coordinating services over which they have control, but may have special difficulty in coordinating long-term care services with services, such as medical care, funded through separate funding streams. However, more information on the advantages and disadvantages of differing structural approaches to organization of care programs will have to await the completion of evaluations of such emerging programs.

Hospice Care

Hospice care has played and will continue to play a special role in the care of persons with AIDS. Hospice was developed primarily for persons with terminal cancer, many of whom are elderly. Hospice care of such individuals has been shown to be cost-effective: while patients receive some services that might otherwise not be received, there are offsetting savings, typically the result of less aggressive medical treatment during the last stages of the dying process. In the National Hospice Study, Mor and his colleagues found that hospice care, by encouraging care out of the hospital, reduced total cost during the last weeks of life (Mor, Greer, & Kastenbaum, 1988).

Hospice care is particularly relevant to the care of persons with AIDS for several reasons. Key to the hospice concept is acceptance of the incurable nature of the disease in the patient in question and the inevitability of the patient's death; this is the rationale for the "care, not cure" hospice philosophy.

At least at the current stage of medical knowledge about AIDS, the disease is virtually universally a terminal illness, although antiviral therapy can extend life. The virtually nonexistent chance of long-term remission, in the present state of medical knowledge, distinguishes it from other diseases that affect significant numbers of nonelderly persons. As such, the "care, not cure" philosophy is particularly appropriate in the care of advanced cases of AIDS. Issues of confronting and dealing with the dying process, previously of concern mostly to gerontologists, have become familiar ones in AIDS care, and again the geriatric care experience has become relevant.

John W. Riley, Jr., has described the hospice approach as one that "facilitates joint decision-making by the dying person and those who are about to become survivors," while helping the dying person to maintain a sense of identity and providing opportunities for emotional expression of feelings by the dying person (Riley & Riley, 1989—and see Chapter 7 in this volume by McKinlay et al.). Hospice care can often better permit dying individuals to negotiate the transition from living to dying, say their farewells, and have their wishes regarding aggressive medical intervention respected. It has traditionally also been an approach that emphasizes adequate medication for pain control, with less emphasis on other concerns of limited relevance to the dying, such as avoidance of addiction.

The original hospice concept—developed by Dr. Cicely Saunders at London's St. Christopher's Hospice—was a residential facility. In the United States, as Riley and Riley (1989) note, hospice care is now typically provided in the patient's home. The hospice home care approach has been described in detail by Martin (1987). Because many persons with AIDS lack housing, particularly among the increasingly significant subpopulation of intravenous drug users with AIDS, residential hospice care is a needed resource in the care system, and the epidemic challenges the hospice movement to provide this "traditional" type of care in addition to hospice home care.

While persons with AIDS have similar needs in many respects to those of the elderly and others who utilize hospice care, there are also significant differences in their needs. Kübler-Ross (1987) points out that, despite the grave ultimate prognosis, the unstable course of AIDS, as compared with most cancers, requires a more flexible model of care than the traditional palliative-care-only regimen, in which the patient is asked to sign a waiver that no active treatment is to be given to prolong life. Without such modification, care might be foregone that could in fact produce months or longer of good-quality life. Other problems with application of the traditional hospice model include the requirement that hospices only admit patients with expected survival of less than 6 months (a requirement that has sometimes but not always been interpreted liberally in the case of persons with AIDS). As in other areas of long-term care, there have been concerns about the reaction of non-AIDS patients and their families to sharing facilities with persons with AIDS. Kübler-Ross asserted in her 1987 book that only 16% of hospices in the United States accepted AIDS patients and that few of them were happy about it, because of concerns about losing financial support from cancer patients and their families. Because of these problems, she concluded that creation of specific hospices specializing in AIDS care is mandatory.

Thus, in the instance of hospice care as in other instances discussed in this chapter, experience gained with other supportive care constituencies is relevant to the care of persons with AIDS, and previous care models can be adapted, but not simply adopted. Mechanical adherence to previously developed models does not adequately address the special needs of PWA. Kübler-Ross's point about the need to modify the traditional hospice care model is reinforced by the work of Jack Little and his associates at the AIDS Project, Los Angeles (Little, Daley, & Fortson, 1987). Reporting on the results of a supportive care project, they note that while virtually all their subjects needed the basic elements of hospice care, such as personal care assistance and help with the emotional aspects of dealing with impending death, only three of 150 subjects elected formal hospice care. Patients were unwilling to forsake aggressive treatments or to accept a prognosis of 6 months or less. Arbitrary screening rules like this 6-month criterion, imposed by third-party payers, need to be modified if useful models such as hospice are to be adequately responsive to the needs of persons with AIDS.

Social and Medical Case Management

Many community-based programs utilize what might be called a "social case management" model, with case managers involving themselves with such matters as benefits entitlement, housing, household maintenance, homemaking, and personal care services. The inclusion of services like private duty nursing and "high-tech home care" into the service package on which case managers draw can further expand the potential management role. A more ambitious model, though one that would be difficult to implement in an environment of separate funding streams, would involve "medical case management," with administrative integration between medical treatment and long-term care. A medical case management model might, for example, involve nurse practitioners who assume responsibility for a whole host of duties, such as working closely with the primary treating physician on the case; adjusting medications under a clinical protocol and with medical backup; seeing the patient both at home and in the clinic; being easily accessible by telephone; providing guidance to the patient, family, and home care personnel on such matters as diet, monitoring side effects of medication, and deciding when symptoms are severe enough to require emergency transportation to the hospital; and being involved in ongoing adjustment of the services package to meet the patient's changing medical status and care needs. Some elements of this model have been incorporated into San Diego's HRSA-funded project for PWA, and some are also in place in several hospital-centered programs for PWA. However, separate funding streams for various components of care, characteristic of the fragmented American health and social care system in general, tend to make such models difficult to implement for PWA, as they have with the elderly population.

A model that offers significant potential not only for linking medical and long-term care management but also for coordinating funding streams is New York State's Designated Center program. This program has potential significance for chronically ill older people as well as for PWA. The provisions of this program, which are summarized in Knickman, Benjamin, and Dunham's (1988) review of case management for persons with AIDS, require participating hospitals to assign a case manager to each patient. Multidisciplinary medical/nursing/mental health/social work teams must be created for planning and coordination of inpatient and outpatient services. This program "bundles" reimbursement for these services with reimbursement for inpatient care, through creation of a higher DRG rate for hospitals that become Designated Centers. This approach could create a strong incentive for hospitals to participate and could establish a single flow of funds that facilitates coordination of services. It could help reduce discontinuity of care and the number of different professionals with whom the patient must interact as he or she moves between hospital and home. The integration of funding streams can have substantial impact on the delivery of home care services for older people (Crystal et al., 1987) and can be expected to have similar impact on care of PWA. While the Designated Center model goes only part of the way in merging funding streams, it is a pragmatic approach that builds on hospital sites that have become, de facto, the principal locus of care for many PWA. It represents a step in the direction of a more coordinated funding pattern. Evaluations of the outcomes and impact of such models are relevant for long-term care of the elderly as well as for planning care for the increasing numbers of PWA.

Coordinated Systems of Care

Even more significant for the future care of both populations may be experiments that go further in merging funding streams by integrating funding for long-term care and for medical care services. In long-term care of older people, the four Social Health Maintenance Organization (SHMO) sites represent a step in this direction of considerable conceptual and structural importance, even though the programs themselves have operated on a relatively small scale, have involved relatively limited long-term care benefits, and have encountered a variety of administrative and financial roadblocks in the course of their implementation (Kane & Kane, 1987; Leutz et al., 1985).

The care of persons with AIDS brings this issue of integration of medical and supportive care to the forefront, providing opportunity for testing models that go further toward funding integration than has been generally feasible with older people. Most PWA are not tied into previously established medical relationships and need to find new sources of specialized medical care in any event. Moreover, it has been estimated that PWA are hospitalized on the average three times a year (Scitovsky & Rice, 1987), providing opportunity for cost savings by community care systems that can eliminate unnecessary hospitalization. Such a model might involve a single capitation payment for total care of PWA (perhaps weighted by some factors such as risk group) that would cover hospitalization, outpatient care, inpatient care, transportation, and other care as needed. A model of this kind would test the hypothesis that a fully coordinated system of care could substantially minimize the need for hospitalization while providing good-quality medical care and maximizing patient satisfaction and quality of life.

Such demonstrations would, in turn, clearly have implications for care of older people as well. As noted, several innovations in the care of PWA have involved developing extensive packages of in-home services largely in order to minimize costly, inappropriate, and unnecessary hospitalization. Research on the costs, outcomes, and implementation experience of such programs could have considerable relevance to the effort to develop less institutionally biased approaches to the care of the chronically ill elderly. Particularly important is assessment of the results and costs of providing so-called "high-tech home care services," such as parenteral nutrition, maintenance of intravenous lines, and respirator care. Such services, increasingly being utilized for older people as the DRG environment leads to hospital discharges "quicker and sicker," have become widespread in care of PWA at home.

EVALUATING THE OUTCOMES OF COMMUNITY-BASED INTERVENTIONS

An important area of convergence in health services research for the aged and for PWA involves evaluation research on the effectiveness and outcomes of community-based long-term care programs. Programs that have been tested to remedy these deficiencies have included a variety of demonstrations, the largest of which, and the most elaborately evaluated, has been the "Channeling" demonstration of national long-term care (Kemper, Brown, Carcagno, et al.,

1986). Despite substantial investments in such evaluations, there has been much disappointment with their results. In part, this has been due to the technical flaws, inconsistency of findings, and general lack of definitiveness of the evaluations. Moreover, even when reliable results *have* been produced, they often have failed to confirm the achievement of at least some of the avowed goals of the demonstrations. There have been problems both of methodology (e.g., do these evaluations fairly measure the effect of the intervention tested?)—and theory (e.g., were the proper questions asked?). As political pressure grows for a national long-term care program for older people, increased attention will be paid to what we do and do not know about the outcomes of community-based long-term care interventions. And as programs for community care of PWA grow, analogous questions will be posed and will need to be answered. A brief overview of some of the major demonstration programs for older people suggests the scope of problems in conducting such evaluations and the inconsistencies in findings based on differing evaluation criteria.

Community-based long-term care demonstration programs for older people have frequently defined their objectives in terms of success in minimizing expenditures on other forms of care, such as hospitals, nursing homes, or other medical care, or in terms of achieving lower total health care costs than would have been incurred had the program not existed. Measured against this economic criterion, many of these programs have failed to demonstrate the intended effect (although another important criterion, quality of life, is often omitted as a measure of success). In a critical review of community-based long-term care demonstration projects, Hughes (1985) concluded that while utilization of noninstitutional services was typically increased, the use of institutional services was usually not substantially reduced. Thus the objective of lower overall health care costs was typically not achieved. Findings from the evaluation of the "Channeling" demonstrations generally are consistent with this pattern. These demonstrations had little or no effect on the use of institutional services and little measurable impact on client health and functioning. However, they did reduce unmet needs reported by clients, increase the use of noninstitutional services, and result in increased client satisfaction with care (Corson et al., 1986; Kemper, Brown, Carcagno, et al., 1986).

Kane and Kane (1987), in a comprehensive review of the literature on long-term care outcomes for older people, similarly conclude that the results of evaluations of community long-term care demonstrations, taken together, have been discouraging. Results on mortality and quality of life have been ambiguous, while effects on use and cost of other services, particularly institutional services, have generally not had the anticipated cost-limiting consequences. However, these studies have also pointed up the difficulty of evaluating long-term care innovations in a real-world environment. Since a variety of services are available from many different sources for "controls" as well as "experimental" program participants, comparison with a true control group is difficult. Where "experimental" demonstration projects are not carefully controlled, comparison or "control" groups may turn out to be higher-functioning or less "service needy" than experimentals, thus falsely making the intervention look as if it had negative effects, or as if its positive effects were offset by other negative consequences.

The substantial, yet frustrating, experience in implementation and evaluation of community care demonstrations for the elderly and the new but growing analogous experience in the context of the care of PWA, suggest that much thought and effort will need to go into the design, implementation, and evaluation of demonstrations in the care of PWA. Although many variations of care models have been tried for older people, few really provide significant integration, either fiscal or administrative, between medical and long-term care. Much can be learned that is relevant to both constituencies by carefully designed evaluation studies of a variety of program and financing models discussed above. Particularly significant would be a test of a fully integrated capitation model with a single funding stream for all medical and long-term care for a defined patient population. This model would draw on the SHMO model, while providing more substantial long-term care services.

As community care programs and long-term care programs for PWA are implemented, methodological issues in their evaluation need to be addressed, and criteria for program success need to be carefully considered. A relevant line of research involves use of quality of well-being assessment as a means of evaluating the overall effect of an intervention or care program. Kaplan and his colleagues (1988) have compared applications of a scale of this type in a population of persons with AIDS and in a principally elderly population with arthritis.

OLDER PEOPLE'S RELATIONSHIPS WITH PERSONS WITH AIDS

There are two major ways in which older people interact directly with PWA in the long-term care system: first, as co-residents in long-term care settings, and second, as informal or formal care providers to PWA.

Patient Commingling and the Fear of Contagion

Fear of contagion has often become an issue when (as noted previously) elderly patients are co-residents, or potential co-residents, with PWA in hospitals or, most especially, in long-term care settings. This fear has been a common theme in battles in various parts of the country over placement of PWA in long-term care facilities and in debates over location of new long-term facilities for PWA. It would be helpful in addressing these issues to have data on the AIDS-related knowledge and attitudes of older people (see the chapter reviewing the relevant literature by Levy & Albrecht in this volume). One source of such information is the special set of supplemental questions on the AIDS-related knowledge and attitudes of the public introduced into the National Health Interview Survey, beginning in August of 1988. Several reports have been issued (National Center for Health Statistics, 1987, 1988a, b), with breakdowns by several variables including ages; unfortunately, the oldest age category was defined as 50+ rather than 60+ or 65+.

Even with this limitation, the data do show that the older respondents were substantially more likely to fear contagion from casual contact. For example, in October 1987, 30% of persons over 50 believed it was "very likely" or "somewhat likely" to get AIDS from using public toilets, 42% from being coughed or sneezed on by someone who has AIDS, 18% from working near someone who has AIDS, 35% from eating in a restaurant where the cook has AIDS, and 11% from shaking hands with or touching someone who has AIDS. These percentages were higher in each case than those for respondents under 50. Given these fears, it is not surprising that older consumers and potential consumers of long-term care would find sharing facilities with PWA unacceptable. Simply being in the same neighborhood with PWA was seen as risky by some. Only 76% of respondents over 50 believed that it is "very unlikely" or "definitely not possible" to get AIDS by living near a hospital or home for AIDS patients (9% thought it "somewhat unlikely," 4% "somewhat" or "very likely," and 10% were "don't knows").

Older People as Care Providers (Formal and Informal)

In addition to encountering the problems of long-term care for persons with AIDS in their role as clients of the long-term care system, older people may also encounter these problems in the capacity of caretakers themselves, either formal or informal. The modal age for PWA is in the thirties, with a not insubstantial number in their forties and beyond. (See the chapter in this volume by Stall, Catania, & Pollack.) As these patients become sicker, they very often fall back on their parents for care—parents who "graduated" from caretaking responsibilities years earlier and who are likely to be elderly themselves. Among patients receiving care from an AIDS care program in New Jersey, for example, 46% were reported to be living with their parents (Kurland, 1988).

These elderly parents of PWA—and, indeed, those elderly parents of PWA whose ill child is not living with them, and those who are grandparents of babies born with the infection—must face special strains. Such stresses may include the direct burden of care; confronting their child's homosexuality or history of drug abuse; coping with social stigma; and dealing with a reversion to caretaking for a dependent child. If the health care and social services systems are to maximize use of the informal support system for care of PWA, the special needs of older parents in this situation need to be better understood.

Another role in which older people may become involved in the problems of care for PWA is as formal care providers. As the supply of direct care personnel becomes tighter in a low unemployment environment, members of the older population are increasingly seen as candidates for recruitment as homemakers and in other paid caretaking roles in long-term care.

Research on family care and on social support more generally for PWA provides an opportunity to improve basic knowledge on these topics. Part of the challenge mandated by the epidemic is to improve our understanding of care-related social support processes, not only among older caretakers, but also among inner-city minorities and other communities often neglected by researchers.

DILEMMAS OF LONG-TERM CARE

Two dilemmas are common to long-term care of both PWA and older people: (1) the short supply of direct care workers and (2) the ethical issues of decision making in terminal cases.

Shortage of Personnel

The issue of supply of direct care workers is one in which the concerns of the elderly and PWA intersect in a variety of ways. These problems are being increasingly reported in several contexts: in hospitals, in nursing homes and other institutional long-term care settings, and in home-care programs.

The crisis in supply of nurses has been widely discussed and could be further exacerbated if private duty nursing is widely used as a home care delivery pattern (as in the example of the AIDS Community Care Alternatives Program discussed above). Increasing problems with the availability of paraprofessional workers, particularly in home-care programs, have received less attention but may also be crucial for the future of long-term care both for older people and for PWA. The supply of workers can be strained by increasing demand and also is vulnerable to external developments; for example, many workers have been undocumented immigrants whose availability is affected by immigration rules (such as the Simpson-Mazzoli legislation). The relatively low-paying jobs in home care compete for workers with hospitals and with jobs outside the health care field. In states like New Jersey, with unemployment in mid-1988 below 4%, agencies experience increasing difficulty in filling positions.

At least into the early 1990s, the total quantity of care required by PWA will be relatively small compared with the scope of care required for the elderly. However, this increment in demand is being added to an already tight supply situation and therefore could become part of a general crisis in the availability of home care, particularly if unemployment remains low. New York became sufficiently concerned with the problem to commission a consultant study of the future demand and supply for home care workers, and increases in real wages and hence in the cost of care are likely to occur in a number of states.

Among unmet AIDS health services research needs is a profile of paid providers of in-home care to PWA. Such research would help in evaluating the extent to which PWA are drawing for in-home care on the same labor pool as older people.

Ethical Issues in Treatment Decisions

Another set of issues familiar in the gerontological context involves medical decision making in terminal care. The classical hospice model involved the acceptance of a terminal care concept that gave priority to patient comfort as opposed to the no-holds-barred effort to treat maximally and sustain every life function to the bitter end. This concept has had considerable influence in AIDS care. However, many unresolved issues of terminal care in the geriatric context, such as controversies about "do-not-resuscitate" or "no-code" orders and guidelines on heroic treatments, remain problems in AIDS care. To what extent is narcotic pain therapy permissible (even, for example, at the cost of addiction or depressing respiratory function, which could speed death)? At what point should a patient have a "no-code" status, and how is this decision to be made? How can the patient's prior wishes properly be taken into account? Despite much philosophical discussion, there is little systematic knowledge as to how such decisions are actually made, what principles providers and caregiving institutions follow in making them, and what are the effects of different terminal care philosophies on such variables as cost or patient comfort.

The question of who can speak for the patient often takes on special difficulty in AIDS cases, where a lover and a parent may both be in the picture. This problem highlights the need to systematize use of advance directives such as living wills or durable powers of attorney, where acceptable to the patient. Research on the impact of advance directives is important both for PWA and for the elderly facing a possible terminal care situation.

Clarification of treatment philosophies, pain management guidelines, and other ethical and human issues of terminal care management is important in long-term care as in hospital care. Providers of long-term care, whether at home or in institutional settings, need help in knowing how to work with patients, their families, and medical personnel on such matters. Too often (as with older people), PWA find themselves in situations in which their care wishes are not followed, because of legal liability concerns, lack of advance planning and guidelines, or other reasons. Better understanding of these problems and development of mechanisms for their resolution are important. Research could identify opportunities for assuring respect for patient wishes concerning care and preventing unnecessary infliction of pain, while conserving health care resources and expenditures for those who can benefit from them.

LONG-TERM CARE OF PWA AND OLDER PEOPLE: COMMONALITY OF THE ISSUES

This chapter, while recognizing that there is some overlap between PWA and old people with longstanding chronic illness, has examined the parallelism between the long-term care needs of the two populations. It has identified certain differences, but also marked similarities, between the two. And it has proposed a common agenda for research and demonstration on improving programs for care of both.

Research needs on this agenda include studies of social support and informal care provision; analyses of use of acute and long-term health care resources by persons with AIDS; research on the outcomes of alternative configurations of long-term care; assessment of the economic and quality-of-care consequences of capitation in the care of PWA; a test of "bundling" funds for medical and long-term care of PWA, along the lines of the Social Health Maintenance Organization demonstrations for older people; and studies on medical care decision making, particularly concerning advance directives and heroic care. Also, studies of the process of psychosocial adaptation to chronic illness, coping with the prospect of death, and the "illness career" of PWA are relevant to both constituencies, and systematic comparisons between the coping processes of elderly and nonelderly chronically ill individuals can shed light on the processes involved in both instances. (See the chapter in this book by McKinlay.)

In addition, we need to understand more about age as a variable among persons with AIDS. Is the process of coping with illness and the utilization of formal and informal care resources different for middle-aged and older persons with AIDS and for younger persons with AIDS? We need to understand more about the role of ethnicity and race in patterns of utilization of long-term care by the chronically ill, including PWA (cf. Greene & Monahan, 1984); these issues are particularly relevant given the severe impact of AIDS in inner-city minority communities, areas which have seldom been the locus of long-term care research in the past. We need methodological studies on measurement of quality of life and outcomes of care that cross the artificial boundaries of age and particular illness. Finally, if we are to move to a more causal understanding of relationships among biological processes, variations in medical care, long-term care provision, social support, and a variety of relevant outcomes (economic, psychological, and medical), we need a research program on the care of persons with AIDS that follows patients longitudinally through the course of illness. Longitudinal research of this kind would serve as a model for addressing key research problems on chronic illness, regardless of the age or diagnosis of the patient.

In sum, the AIDS epidemic has brought new attention and urgency to many longstanding problems and irrationalities in the long-term care system. It has led to a range of new service delivery demonstrations and models in the AIDS care context. Earlier research on long-term care has much relevance to the care of PWA. Conversely, the development and evaluation of new models for care of PWA could provide lessons for improving long-term care for the elderly.

REFERENCES

Bloom, David E., and Geoffrey Carliner. 1988. "The Economic Impact of AIDS in the United States." *Science* 239:604–610.

Caplan, Ronald. forthcoming. "The Cost of Caring for Intravenous Drug-Related AIDS Cases in New Jersey." *Journal of Drug Issues.*

Corson, W., T. Granneman, N. Holdens, and C. Thornton. 1986. *Channeling Effects on Formal Community-Based Services and Housing.* Plainsboro, NJ: Mathematica Policy Research.

Crystal, Stephen. 1984. *America's Old Age Crisis: Public Policy and the Two Worlds of Aging* (rev. ed.). New York: Basic Books.

Crystal, Stephen, Camilla Flemming, Pearl Beck, and Geraldine Smolka. 1987. *The Management of Home Care Services.* New York: Springer Publishing Co.

Crystal, Stephen, and Marguerite Jackson. 1988a. "The Hidden Epidemic: Public Policy and the Care of Persons with AIDS-Related Complex." *AIDS Patient Care* 2(4):4–7.

Crystal, Stephen, and Marguerite Jackson. 1988b. "Psychosocial Adaptation and Economic Circumstances of Persons with Acquired Immunodeficiency Syndrome and Persons with AIDS-Related Complex." Working Paper. New Brunswick, NJ: Institute for Health, Health Care Policy, and Aging Research, Rutgers University. Forthcoming in *Family and Community Health.*

Feder, J., and William Scanlon. 1980. "Regulating the Bed Supply in Nursing Homes." *Milbank Memorial Fund Quarterly* 58:54–88.

Grant, Igor, J. Atkinson, J.R. Hesselink, Caroline J. Kennedy, Douglas Richman, Stephen Spector, and J. Allan McCutchan. 1987. "Evidence for Early Central Nervous System Involvement in the Acquired Immune Deficiency Syndrome and Other Human Immunodeficiency Virus Infections." *Annals of Internal Medicine* 107:828–836.

Greene, V.L., and J.J. Monahan. 1984. "Comparative Utilization of Community Based Long-Term Care Services by Hispanic and Anglo Elderly in a Case Management System." *Journal of Gerontology* 39:730–735.

Hay, Joel W., Dennis H. Osmond, and Mark A. Jacobson. 1988. *Projecting the Medical Costs of AIDS and ARC in the United States.* Paper presented at the Fourth International Conference on AIDS, Stockholm.

Hing, Esther. 1987. "The Use of Nursing Homes by the Elderly: Preliminary Data from the 1985 National Nursing Home Survey." *Advance Data from Vital and Health Statistics,* No. 311. Hyattsville, MD: National Center for Health Statistics.

Hughes, S.L. 1985. "Apples and Oranges: A Critical Review of Evaluations of Community-Based Long-Term Care." *Health Services Research* 20:461–488.

Kane, Rosalie, and Robert Kane. 1987. *Long-Term Care: Principles, Programs, and Practices.* New York: Springer Publishing Co.

Kaplan, Robert M., John P. Anderson, Albert Wu, William Christopher Mathews, Franklin Kozin, and David Orenstein. 1988. "The Quality of Well-Being Scale: Applications in AIDS, Cystic Fibrosis, and Arthritis." Paper prepared for Henry J. Kaiser Family Foundation Advances in Health Status Assessment Conference; forthcoming in *Medical Care.*

Kemper, Peter, R.S. Brown, G.J. Carcagno, et al. 1986. *The Evaluation of the National Long-Term Care Demonstration: Final Report.* Plainsboro, NJ: Mathematical Policy Research.

Kizer, K.W., J. Rodriguez, and G.G. McHolland. 1987. *An Updated Quantitative Analysis of AIDS in California.* Sacramento, CA: California Department of Health Services, April.

Knickman, James R., A.E. Benjamin, and Nancy Dunham. 1988. *Case Management for Persons with AIDS: Existing Models and Research Issues.* Paper presented at the annual meeting of the Association for Health Services Research, San Francisco, June 27.

Kübler-Ross, Elisabeth. 1987. *AIDS: The Ultimate Challenge.* New York: Macmillan.

Kurland, Carol. 1988. *New Jersey's AIDS Community Care Alternatives Program.* Presentation at meetings of New Jersey Chapter, National Association of Social Workers, Morristown, NJ, March 25.

Leutz, W.N., J.N. Greenberg, R. Abrahams, J. Prottas, L.M. Diamond, and L. Gruenberg, 1985. *Changing Health Care for an Aging Society.* Lexington, MA: Lexington Books.

Little, Jack, Steve Daley, and Howard Fortson. 1987. *AIDS Home Health, Attendant or Hospice Care Pilot Study.* Los Angeles: AIDS Project Los Angeles.

Martin, Jeannee. 1987. "Sustaining Care for Persons with AIDS." In *The Person with AIDS: Nursing Perspectives,* edited by Jerry D. Durham and Felissa Cohen. New York: Springer Publishing Co.

Mor, Vincent, David S. Greer, and Robert Kastenbaum. 1988. *The Hospice Experiment.* Baltimore: Johns Hopkins University Press.

National Academy of Sciences, Institute of Medicine, 1986. *Confronting AIDS: Directions for Public Health, Health Care, and Research.* Washington, DC: National Academy Press.

National Center for Health Statistics. 1987. "AIDS Knowledge and Attitudes, Provisional Data from the National Health Interview Survey: United States, August 1987." *Vital and Health Statistics* No. 146, November 19.

National Center for Health Statistics. 1988a. "AIDS Knowledge and Attitudes, Provisional Data from the National Health Interview Survey: United States, September 1987." *Vital and Health Statistics* No. 148, January 18.
National Center for Health Statistics. 1988b. "AIDS Knowledge and Attitudes, Provisional Data from the National Health Interview Survey: United States, October 1987." *Vital and Health Statistics* No. 150, March 9.
New Brunswick Home News. 1988. "Angry Mob Protests Allocating 120 AIDS Beds at Nursing Home." April 2, A10.
Riley, Matilda White, and John W. Riley, Jr., eds. 1989. *The Quality of Aging: Strategies for Interventions.* Special issue of *The Annals* (May).
Scanlon, William. 1980. "A Theory of the Nursing Home Market." *Inquiry* 17(2):25–41.
Scitovsky, Ann, and Dorothy Rice. 1987. "Estimates of the Direct and Indirect Costs of Acquired Immunodeficiency Syndrome in the United States, 1985, 1986, and 1991." *Public Health Reports* 102(1):5–17.
Straham, Genevieve. 1987. "Nursing Home Characteristics: Preliminary Data from the 1985 National Nursing Home Survey." *Advance Data from Vital and Health Statistics,* No. 131. Hyattsville, MD: National Center for Health Statistics.
U.S. Senate Special Committee on Aging. 1986. *Developments in Aging, 1985.* Report No. 99-242. Washington, DC: Government Printing Office.

PART IV

Societal Consequences

CHAPTER 9

Forecasting the Impact of the AIDS Epidemic on Elderly Populations

Kenneth G. Manton and Burton Singer

The AIDS epidemic has seriously impacted many different population categories in the United States (e.g., IV drug users, gay and bisexual men, minority group members, and people receiving blood transfusions, including those with hemophilia). A population category that, to date, has not been widely recognized as significantly affected is the nation's elderly. Yet unfortunately there are signs that the impact of AIDS on this segment will become increasingly important. On the one hand, the numbers of older people afflicted with the disease are likely to increase. Not only are the elderly especially vulnerable to the HIV virus because they have higher risks of chronic diseases and physiological impairments; in addition, the potency of the human immune system itself tends to decline with age. On the other hand, the projected rise in the health service demands of younger AIDS patients will create competition with frail older people for scarce health care resources, thereby indirectly threatening the general health of the old. (See the chapter by Crystal in this volume.)

Despite the predictable course of the AIDS epidemic in the elderly population, no accurate quantitative measures of this impact are currently available. The purpose of this chapter, then, is to establish a research agenda for forecasting (1) both quantitative and qualitative aspects of the future course of the AIDS epidemic among older adults, (2) the impact of increased AIDS-related demand for acute and long-term health care services on the access to and availability of such health services to the elderly; and (3) the compilation and collection of data necessary to make such forecasts.

This paper was produced with funds from the Behavioral and Social Research Program of the National Institute on Aging; no funds from any AIDS research program were employed in its preparation.

REQUIREMENTS OF FORECASTING MODELS

A number of forecasts have already been made of the future course of the AIDS epidemic. However, forecasts are made for many purposes using many different types of models. One type of forecast is the short-term extrapolation of recent trends in the change of event rates, for example, extrapolations based on the last 5 years of the rate of change of the prevalence of AIDS in the U.S. population (Brookmeyer & Mitchell, 1986; Morgan & Curran, 1986). Over relatively short periods of time for processes with as much "inertia" as the trend of a national epidemic of a chronic disease process with a lengthy latency period, such projections may give good "order of magnitude" estimates of the number of cases that will both emerge and require significant amounts of health services. This type of projection strategy is used by the U.S. Public Health Service to estimate the number of AIDS cases for 1992 (and more recently 1993).

Such simple extrapolation projection techniques are useful in helping to sensitize both the public and policy makers to the magnitude of the societal problems that must be faced to cope effectively with the AIDS epidemic. We argue, however, that such simple projections have only limited utility for evaluating:

1. the effects of specific public health intervention programs to control disease incidence,
2. the effects of treatment programs on survival and the implications of changes in survival for future health resource requirements, and
3. possible changes in the behavior of the disease process in specific subpopulations with particular exposure and biological characteristics.

We further argue that to produce projections that will deal satisfactorily with these problems, it is necessary to develop forecasting models that meet three criteria: that is, the models must (1) be *biosocially* realistic, (2) appropriately represent the *uncertainty* of the phenomena to be described, and (3) be able to integrate data from *multiple sources.*

In this chapter we address what each of these three characteristics of forecasts implies, and we discuss two concrete areas of applications that illustrate the principles involved. Detailed data to estimate parameters directly in many of the more fine-grained, biosocially motivated models that we discuss are not currently available and are unlikely to be available in the near future. In this situation, we feel that model development is of the utmost importance and that its role is to integrate the wide variety of data available on the clinical, epidemiological, and social dimensions of HIV infection and expression of AIDS in a coherent mathematical and statistical framework. We feel that such models should be used to answer "what if" questions under a variety of assumed scenarios for the parameters. Indeed, there seems to be no alternative to the full range of model development discussed below if one is to have a comprehensive logical framework at hand for understanding the diverse and complex facets of the AIDS epidemic.

BIOSOCIALLY REALISTIC MODELS

The requirement that the model employed in forecasting be "biosocially realistic" means that the mathematical structure of the model used to describe the processes generating the morbid and lethal events of interest be representative of the available empirical and theoretical evidence on the biological, as well as the social and epidemiological, nature of the disease phenomena. Several dimensions must be evaluated in order to determine whether the structure of a model is both biologically and sociobehaviorally realistic.

Nature of the Disease Process

The first dimension to be evaluated is that the mathematical model well approximate the behavior of the disease process at the level of the individual human organism and, with appropriate data, at levels of biological organization below that of the human organism. Additionally, in the case of infectious processes, one must appropriately model at a higher level the "between-individual" modes of transmission, that is, construct a model of how the infectious agent enters the physiological system of the organism (Anderson et al., 1986; Dietz, 1988; Hethcote & Yorke, 1983; May & Anderson, 1987). Such modeling is particularly important for AIDS because of its complex natural history within the body. Specifically, some estimates suggest that about 35% of HIV-positive persons will manifest formal symptoms of AIDS within 8 years of infection. Thus, in contrast to many other types of infectious disease processes, the biological latency period for AIDS is extremely long.

Not only is the period of latency lengthy, but it appears to be strongly affected by a number of host characteristics. For example, the latent period can be affected by recreational drug use, stress, co-morbid infectious processes, and other physiological and behavioral factors affecting the immune system (Ho, Pomerantz, & Kaplan, 1987). Indeed, one model of AIDS activation suggests that certain types of infectious processes stimulate the immune system and, by this stimulation, produce biochemical effects that result in activation of the latent AIDS virus (which may be more often present in macrophages than T-cells) (Ho et al., 1987). Such stimulation of the immune system by other infections (or perhaps even by attempts to immunize the individual with a vaccine) thus may be a necessary "triggering" phenomena in the manifestation of AIDS.

Consequently, it has been suggested that alteration of life-style (i.e., toward adopting a number of health-promoting behaviors—better nutrition, avoidance of other infections, better primary health care) may delay the occurrence of triggering infections and may leave the immune system intact, thereby significantly extending the latent period (Ho et al., 1987). Obviously these life-style modifications are more likely among, say, middle-class, highly educated, gay men than they are in the IV drug use population. They also suggest that such behavior modification may delay the onset of the disease to later in the life course, where the age-related decline of the immune system below some threshold efficacy may be the triggering event.

Parenthetically, efforts at developing forecasting models that are based upon the physiology of the natural history of the disease process in the individual may have importance far beyond that of AIDS itself, because other "slow" viral infections are probably an important factor for a number of prevalent neoplastic and autoimmune disorders. For example, slow viruses have been implicated in certain types of lymphomas, leukemia, and liver, cervical, and breast cancers (Haywood, 1986). Autoimmune responses triggered by reaction to slow viruses have been proposed as the initiating mechanism for polymyositis, some subtypes of Alzheimer's disease, multiple sclerosis, rheumatoid arthritis, diabetes (Type I), and other chronic degenerative diseases (Haywood, 1986).

It may be that to adequately assess the impact on the elderly population of many chronic degenerative disease processes it will be necessary to develop similar types of infectious process models with long latencies (e.g., where the long latencies occur because a virus remains dormant in the DNA of certain cell populations until age-related changes in the immune system or stress from other chronic diseases allows it to emerge). We, for example, do not know what the long-term public health implication of nearly universal immunization for polio and other childhood diseases will be or what the effects of new vaccines for diseases such as hepatitis B will imply for long-term health trends. Thus, we expect that this type of long-term forecast, involving terms reflecting "genetic" drift of the virus of chronic infections and chronic physiological response to viral infection, will be increasingly important in public health planning in the future. Biologically appropriate models can be made extremely sensitive to the earliest signs of such emergent (though currently unrecognized) epidemics.

The fundamental point may be that we should not view the AIDS epidemic as an aberration, or an isolated event, but possibly a result of natural biological processes that will periodically cause new diseases to emerge (and some old ones to possibly disappear). There is considerable epidemiological and biological evidence to support this view (Haywood, 1986), such as the fact that the virulence of the plague in the late Middle Ages may have been eventually limited by genetic shifts in the infectious agent, the fact that rheumatoid arthritis did not appear to exist in England in the Middle Ages but apparently evolved in the 1700's from a virus affecting animals, and, in the short term, the cyclical change in influenza viruses, the emergence of AIDS itself, and the more recent evidence on emergence of viruses related to AIDS—these latter viruses also with rapid rates of genetic drift.

These issues are of particular interest in studying the impact of viruses on older people because, with their weakened immune response, older people represent organisms that bear a unique relation to the genetic evolutionary processes of viral infectious agents: that is, the vulnerabilities of old age did not emerge directly from the long-term evolutionary change of the species but are, to a considerable degree, a result of recent and complex sociomedical, economic, and environmental factors.

Heterogeneity of Disease Processes

The total prevalence of AIDS in the United States population is not monolithic: it is clearly generated by a mix of heterogeneous disease processes operating in different ways in subpopulations with different co-morbid and risk conditions. As a consequence, a model that fails to represent the changing mix of such different processes in subpopulations cannot accurately predict the long-term impact of the disease process on the population as a whole; nor can such a model accurately represent the effects of different types of interventions. Thus, a second necessary feature of a biosocially realistic model is that it correctly relates the operation of heterogeneous disease processes in different individuals to the average incidence and prevalence rates in the total population. Many standard infectious disease models of epidemics do not represent such heterogeneity (Bailey, 1975); however, this situation is changing rapidly in response to the challenge of understanding AIDS and sexually transmitted diseases (STDs) generally (Halloran & Struchiner, 1988; Hethcote & Yorke, 1983; Pickering et al., 1986).

Multidimensionality of the Disease

Another aspect of projections that require biosocially realistic models is the necessity of anticipating future qualitative stages of the disease epidemic. Specifically, one reservoir of the AIDS virus in the human body is the central nervous system (CNS). This reservoir has been evidenced in the manifestation of subacute encephalitis (AIDS dementia complex) (Ho et al., 1987). Since it is suspected that the latent period for AIDS might be as much as 10 to 15 years, or even longer in some individuals, there is a serious question whether much of the latent AIDS infection may first become manifest in an increased incidence of relatively early onset dementia in the future. A biologically realistic model could help evaluate the likelihood and magnitude of such dementia emerging in more elderly HIV-infected persons in the future.

The emergence or nonemergence of dementia reflects a third factor for modeling the AIDS epidemic. That is, that the manifestation of AIDS is "multidimensional," with the manifestation of the disease in a particular host being a function of the physiological state of the host. Thus, even when simply counting AIDS cases there has been considerable debate over what to count (i.e., over the precise definition of an AIDS case) and how to reflect the disease burden of the AIDS-associated opportunistic infections (formerly designated as ARC). With very long-term infections possibly affecting the elderly, this becomes particularly difficult where the lethal processes for many chronic diseases may be significantly accelerated by an independent but concomitant HIV infection. An example of a similar phenomenon is the fact that the contribution of Alzheimer's disease to mortality at advanced ages (or the effect of osteoporosis on mortality mediated by intervening accidental events) was only recently identified as a major public health problem (Katzman, 1986). Indeed, it can be argued that, like Alzheimer's disease, few people are killed outright by the primary disease process but typically die of multiple, co-morbid infections and neoplastic processes to which the AIDS infection has made the individual susceptible. This argues that a simple "case counting" approach to measuring the progression of the epidemic, especially if treatment significantly prolongs survival (so that persons survive longer in a chronic debilitated state with many co-morbid conditions), may not be adequate for planning for health services. Models of such complex functional and disease states have been developed for elderly and oldest-old populations (Berkman, Singer, & Manton, 1989; Manton et al., 1987) but have not yet been applied to the clinical status and mortality of AIDS sufferers and HIV-infected persons.

Duration of the Disease Process

A fourth aspect of a biosocially realistic model that could help improve the accuracy of health services forecasts requires better representations of duration. The models should allow improved representation of (1) the duration of different stages of the disease process (and the impact of treatment on those durations); and (2) the total requirement for health resources where the specific set of services required at different disease stages could be weighted by the duration (current, and as projected under a given treatment intervention) of those stages. Examples of this type of phenomena are the potential for higher prevalence rates of AIDS, even given lower incidence rates, due to improved survival. Some clinical trial results suggest that treatment with AZT may cause a four- to sixfold reduction in mortality rates after 9 months (Fischl et al., 1987). One study in New York City suggests that, with adequate medical care, the survival time for persons with AIDS may be 8 years or longer

(Rothenberg et al., 1988). Other treatments of major complicating conditions (e.g., of specific types of pneumonia often associated with HIV infection) may also significantly improve survival (e.g., the treatment of Pneumocystis carinii by pentamidine, trimethotrexate, trimethoprim, and sulfamethone) (Hughes, 1987). The use of AZT earlier in the infection and the use of combined chemotherapeutic protocols (e.g., sequential AZT and DDC) may also significantly lengthen survival. Indeed, the National Cancer Institute has suggested that, insofar as approval procedures can be streamlined by the Food and Drug Administration, treatments may be available in the near future that will allow the long term management of AIDS in much the same way as diabetes or hypertension may be controlled over the life course. All of these improvements in survival will be purchased by dramatically higher treatment costs over longer periods of time. Accurate forecasts and simulations of the health services required to deal with AIDS will require biologically detailed modeling that reflects such contingencies.

An additional area where a biosocially realistic model may improve our ability to forecast service needs is the effort to alter the future mix of services provided to AIDS sufferers. For example, it appears that much more of AIDS treatment, at least at certain stages in the disease process, could occur on an outpatient basis—or in long term care institutions (Weinberg & Murray, 1987). The investigation of the use of long-term care as alternative service options for AIDS patients was a recommendation of the 1988 presidential AIDS study commission. To know how much service patterns could be altered, one needs again to model realistically the duration and qualitative characteristics of different stages in the disease process: for example, the level of functional disability in different stages of the disease process, the set of associated co-morbid conditions, and the intrinsic physiological status of the patient (e.g., if the patient has good or bad cardiopulmonary status). Further, there will be a need to collect data specifically on the little-studied issue of the ways in which current long-term care services could be useful to AIDS patients, and how they might need to be adapted to treat these patients. For example, for AIDS patients certain nursing services currently provided by home health agencies would have to be modified with respect to sterile and reverse isolation procedure—especially with home health workers possibly moving from AIDS sufferers to impaired elderly in poor health. Moreover, there are issues of access, involving the willingness of current long-term care service providers to treat AIDS patients.

REPRESENTATION OF UNCERTAINTY

In addition to biosocially realistic models, the second major requirement for improved forecasting technology is the development of techniques to appropriately represent the uncertainty of the phenomena to be described. In one example of the importance of this requirement, the New York City Health Department released estimates of the number of New Yorkers infected with HIV as 200,000—half of the 400,000 figure that had been previously used by the city (Lambert, 1988). These numbers were in conflict not only with the city's prior estimates but also with other studies arguing that the prior city estimates were underestimates. The release of the new projections may have caused a strong reaction because to date there are few estimates of the statistical uncertainty of any set of AIDS projections, so that each estimate tends to be taken literally as a so-called "point estimate." In fact, each of these projections may fall within the window of uncertainty associated with the forecasts because of the compounding of errors in a number of different data sources and the failure to explicitly model these measurement errors when making estimates.

One aspect of the characterization of the uncertainty of a forecast interacts with the development of a realistic model of the biosocial processes involved. If the biosocial processes are not adequately described, then the total variation of the events to be described cannot be accurately decomposed into "deterministic" and "stochastic" components. If the stochastic component of the total variation is not accurately estimated, then (1) incorrect inferences will be made about the statistical validity of estimates of different features of the process, and (2) the uncertainty of future forecasts cannot be ascertained. An example of where such phenomena are important is where a model is "overfit" to the data, that is, features of the data that result from chance variation are mistakenly integrated into the mathematical structure of the forecasting model. Such an overfit model can, potentially, produce serious bias in long-term forecasts. Such overfitting is a frequent occurrence in the analysis of data on biosocial processes and is a direct result of using generic, statistical models without a clear theoretical specification of the processes one is attempting to model.

Basically, one can always trivially "fit" or "explain" all of the variation within a given set of data using standard "generic" statistical models. Such a model, however, when used to forecast beyond the limits of the data, will produce forecasts that include, and likely amplify, the chance elements in the data. The only guard against this serious source of forecast error is biosocially based specification of one's model. Then when forecast errors arise, the deviation between predictions and actual events will tend to be interpretable in biological, epidemiological, and behavioral terms and will suggest further refinements of the original model. Such monitoring of forecast results, using the feedback to constantly adapt the model to new information on trends in disease behavior, is a necessary aspect of both making and properly utilizing forecasts. These forecasts are to be viewed as important tools to understanding the disease process at both the individual and population level. It is naive to view forecasting as a one-time effort at predicting the magnitude of the public health problem of AIDS at some future fixed date. This is more a "race track" than a scientific view of the utility of modeling for forecasting.

Another important area of model development is appropriately representing stochasticity to (1) describe how uncertainty behaves as data are aggregated or disaggregated, and (2) how uncertain are rates based on small numbers of cases (such as occurs in the mapping of the prevalence of cases in local areas) and where there are real differences in disease risk between areas and between individuals within areas. This type of problem emerges in one of the examples discussed below, where AIDS prevalence is mapped for the United States. The basic point is that the grouping of individuals within areas is generally based upon the use of geographic boundaries determined by administrative convenience (e.g., states, counties, State Economic Areas, census tracts). In order to map the data in a way that reflects the variation of the processes (of both onset and progression) over individuals and subpopulations one must have a model that appropriately relates the event rates at the aggregated level with the processes at the individual level (i.e., that, after adjusting for stochasticity, the subarea rates recompose to yield the national rates no matter what level of decomposition is used). Clearly, the development of a model that has the appropriate properties under the operations of aggregation and disaggregation is mathematically difficult (see Manton et al., 1987, 1989, for example). This type of "closure" under the operation of aggregation is not a property of most analytic strategies currently employed in the analysis of zero prevalence data. Consequently, the current maps of AIDS prevalence must be viewed with considerable caution (Centers for Disease Control, 1987; Curran et al., 1988), as must the age-, race-, and neighborhood-specific maps of HIV incidence—such as those released in 1988 for New York City.

INTEGRATION OF DATA FROM MULTIPLE SOURCES

The third major area of forecasting methodology that needs to be developed is that of integrating data from multiple sources and of different types. Logical and consistent integration of different sets of data depends, of course, upon the two previously described requisites: biosocially realistic models must have been used, particularly if findings on different stages of the disease are to be gleaned from different studies; and appropriate models of uncertainty and selectivity bias must have been used with the different observational plans used to generate the data.

Need for Integration of Multiple-Source Data

It is our view that models that can integrate data from various sources will be a necessity in studying and forecasting the AIDS epidemic because, though there are a large number of studies on AIDS, they generally are limited in scope, population coverage, and time (Centers for Disease Control, 1987; and see the chapter in this volume on methodological considerations by Levy & Albrecht). To effectively use this large fixed investment in existing data, the analytic models employed must be able to recognize and deal with this diversity. We also are quite pessimistic about the cost-effectiveness of investment in large nationally representative surveys of seroprevalence, disease incidence and prevalence, and disease processes. This is because the disease mechanism is too complex, its population incidence too low, and the privacy and confidentiality issues too great to allow such surveys of infection to be successful. The only national surveys that are likely to be fruitful are those that capture dimensions of behaviors and attitudes toward risk taking and service use relevant to infection treatment or management of the disease. To evaluate the biosocial parameters of the epidemic, both at an individual and population level, it seems far more cost-effective (and likely more scientifically valid) if (1) the existing large volume of data is evaluated with appropriate analytic models, (2) areas of critical, high-priority data gaps are identified, and (3) small, highly targeted, well-designed, and focused studies are conducted to fill those gaps. Likewise, if the operation of the infectious disease process can be modeled for representative individuals from different subpopulations, then an appropriate "mixing" model (i.e., model of the population distribution of each of the different types of individuals) can help integrate results from studies of "select," well-defined populations.

In addition, different "observational" plans (sampling schedules over time, space, and stage of process) are associated with different types of stochastic processes, which determine the distribution of outcomes of events due to random factors. With the uncertainty in each of the different types of observational plan well characterized, it is possible to develop models of uncertainty for the integrated set of data. This type of integration of sources of stochasticity will depend heavily on what is referred to as "super-population" theory, which assigns a more limited role to stochasticity in the sampling process and a greater emphasis on developing appropriate models of the event-generating process (including the processes by which data are generated) that is assumed to underlie the data generated from multiple observational plans.

With a biosocially realistic model of the basic health process of interest *and* a defensible characterization of the stochasticity intrinsic to the phenomena and the data collection plan, one will be able to determine how uncertainty of various types propagates through the projections. Specifically, error in model specification will propagate directly (e.g., as a fixed mean square error). Stochasticity due to sampling variability will propagate quadratically. Stochasticity due to the operation of the underlying event process will propagate linearily. The cumulative effect of each of these sources of error will determine the forecasting horizon that is possible with a given model: that is, the rate at which the information contained in the parameters of the model is overwhelmed by the propagation of the uncertainty in the forecasts will determine how far in the future the forecasts will remain informative. Though such forecasting "horizons" are well recognized in the physical sciences (e.g., in meteorology), such issues are seldom systematically dealt with in epidemiological and demographic forecasts. (For an exception, see Manton, 1987; Yashin et al., 1987, 1988, where the bounds to forecast the health and mortality of human populations are discussed for several classes of multivariate models of physiological systems.)

An understanding of models that can successfully integrate data also has important implications for the design of data collection strategies. That is, because of resource and other constraints (e.g., ethical constraints on the degree of intrusion in an individual's life; the disruptive effects of measurement on the phenomena), compromises must always be made in data collection design. Given the distribution of the epidemic, with high concentration in subpopulations difficult to both identify and interview (e.g., IV drug users), the problem of assessing the total impact of AIDS on the entire U.S. population is quite difficult. But a substantial improvement over the effort to date is feasible. Techniques for the design of data collection can be influenced by concepts from "optimal" design to identify the specific areas where gaps in knowledge are the greatest and how resources should be distributed to increase most effectively the information about the process.

Integrating Data from Regional and Local Estimates

Of central importance for forecasting the impact of the AIDS epidemic on the elderly population, then, is an understanding of HIV seroprevalence and AIDS incidence rates over both time and space. The spatial aspect is particularly critical because of the very uneven national distribution—among and within cities and regions—of health care facilities and properly trained personnel to deal with current and potential future demand for services by HIV-positive persons and AIDS cases.

Although seroprevalence maps at various levels of geographic refinement (Centers for Disease Control, 1987; Curran et al., 1988; Lambert, 1988) have been produced to date, inconsistencies and considerable variation even in point estimates for the same location result from the very heterogeneous nature of the populations on which the rate estimates are based. In one instance, neighborhood-specific maps of HIV infection rates by age and race were based primarily on an analysis of blood samples taken mainly from mothers and infants—even though men are believed to have much higher incidence rates (Lambert, 1988). In principle these disparities could be resolved by national and regional random samples; however, the rates of compliance with blood testing that would be essential for the success of such ventures, given the low prevalence rate of HIV infection (variously estimated at less than 1%) and the accompanying confidentiality problems, raise doubts about the practicality of large population surveys, as previously discussed. Alternatively, regional seroprevalence rates can be produced by combining estimates from a multiplicity of special—in most instances—convenience samples in which voluntary self-selection plays a central role in defining the surveyed population. The full range of strategies and judgments that are necessary to produce defensible small area seroprevalence estimates can be illustrated with a simple example. We present this admittedly idealized prototype as a stimulus to AIDS researchers to pursue the production of seroprevalence maps at the refined level that has already been achieved, for example, for cancer mortality maps (Riggan et al., 1987).

Consider a geographical region containing one (or several) sexually transmitted disease (STD) clinics and a gay population that is the target of a seroprevalence survey with very tightly controlled confidentiality for respondents. Our aim is to estimate the seroprevalence rate for the region using STD surveillance and gay survey data alone. This is the simplest prototypical setting for geographic seroprevalence rate estimation that still contains the essential features of more complex settings often involving 10 or more different kinds of data bases.

Figure 9.1 provides a graphical representation of the population structure of a region in which STD clinics are available for voluntary entry and in which a seropositivity survey of homosexuals with voluntary compliance is being conducted. The STD clinics actually provide seroprevalence rates conditional on the individuals at least suspecting some STD (which may be, for example, only gonorrhea) *and* voluntary self-selection into the clinic. The survey recovers a seroprevalence rate conditional on identification as gay *and* voluntary agreement to participate in seropositivity testing. These conditional rates, even if they are based on large numbers of cases, must be combined with the probability of voluntary self-selection to visit an STD clinic among the STD-infected population, the probability that a gay man has an STD, the fraction of the region population that is identified as gay, the fraction of STD cases in the nonhomosexual population, and the probability of compliance among gays surveyed in order to produce a defensible regional seroprevalence rate. In the Appendix to this chapter we present a formal decomposition of the regional rate into these components. However, the essential qualitative point is that separate empirical estimates of the

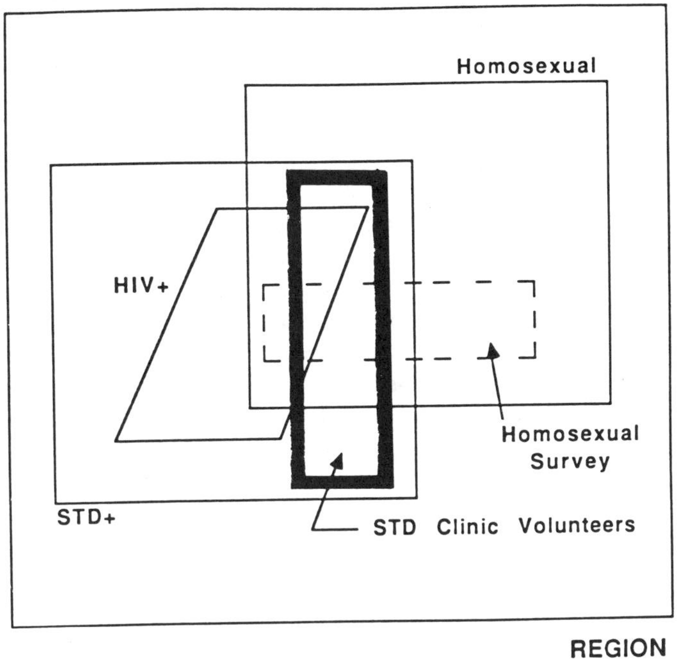

FIGURE 9.1 Schematic view of a region whose seroprevalence rate is to be estimated from convenience samples, selection probabilities, and other indirect evidence.

voluntary self-selection probabilities (or educated guesses of them) play an essential role in the calculation of an overall regional rate. Providing a clear rationale for self-selection probabilities is an important challenge that must be met if we are to have any kind of reliable picture of the impact of HIV transmission on the demand for health care.

In addition to difficulties of obtaining selection probabilities, the basic rates estimated from STD clinics and/or a single survey of gays can be very unstable due to the small number of positive cases. The chance occurrence or nonoccurrence of a single case can have a disproportionate effect on the rate estimate for a condition that is relatively rare in the overall population. Such statistical instability makes the identification of very small but important rates difficult and tends to conceal patterns by masking clusters of risk groups and/or local areas (or clinics) that may in fact have similar rates. We increase the stability of raw local area rates (e.g., those from two or three neighborhood STD clinics) by borrowing information from a larger, more coarsely defined—but nevertheless similar—aggregate population (Manton et al.,

1989; Riggan et al., 1987) and combining it with the local rate(s). The substantive arguments that defend the claim of "*similar* aggregate population" provide the rationale for interpreting the stabilized rates as more trustworthy indicators of local area rates than the raw observed rates.

Formal details of "information borrowing" (or empirical Bayes) strategies, as they pertain to geographic rate estimation, are presented in Riggan et al. (1987) and Manton et al. (1989). The central point for the present discussion is to emphasize that the stabilized rates for STD clinics alone, homosexual surveys alone, et cetera, are essential, but by no means the only, adjustments of raw local area (or single source) seroprevalence rates required to produce an overall unbiased area-specific rate. The self-selection probabilities mentioned above, and formally defined in the Appendix, are critical components of any defensible area-specific rates. Special population surveys (e.g., of IV drug users) aimed at ascertaining reasonable bounds for the self-selection probabilities are, in our opinion, important for providing the most basic guidance in forecasting the likely increases in numbers of HIV-positive persons, AIDS cases, and the resultant increases in demand for health care.

LONG-RANGE POPULATION FORECASTING

In addition to the use of selection probabilities and empirical Bayes adjusted convenience sample rates to study the geographic variability of the HIV infection and its concentration in certain defined "at-risk" populations, it will be necessary to develop much-improved long-range population forecasting models. The currently employed models are largely descriptive in that they are often based on biosocially naive assumptions about the effect of the disease on the individual level. Hence it is generally not possible to use those models for a number of important planning and scientific functions. Models with quite different structures will be required. Below we describe three types of projection models that must be developed to fulfill the range of tasks for which forecasts and simulations will be required (as outlined above).

Models of Health Service Impact

A very important use of forecasting models will be to project future population requirements for health services due to the impact of AIDS. To do this appropriately we need quite different models than have been employed to date. Such models must minimally (1) describe the numbers and duration of residence in several AIDS-related health states (e.g., noninfected; HIV-infected but latent;

early disease manifestation; fully developed AIDS but treatable; death from AIDS; death from other causes but HIV-infected; death from other causes but not HIV-infected); (2) relate rates of transition between HIV-related health states to observable covariates and to the potential sources of unobservable heterogeneity; and (3) stratify states, transition rates, and covariates by the specific identity of major at risk populations. Such models have already been successfully used in modeling the impact of chronic diseases on the U.S. population (Manton et al., 1989; Manton & Stallard, 1987). These models employ modeling strategies called "stochastic compartment modeling," whereby the identity of states, and the form of the temporal dependency of the transition rates between states, is specified on the basis of biosocial theory and evidence from ancillary studies. Microsimulation models focusing on HIV transmission in heterogeneous populations are beginning to appear (Bongaarts, 1987); however, the requisite within-individual detail—essential for health service assessment—has not been incorporated to date.

A model with this much detail provides a series of strategies for including information from a number of different studies on different aspects of the disease process and in different risk groups. For example, one may adopt purely Bayesian techniques, use joint likelihood approaches with the missing information principle or an engineering simulation approach. It also provides the necessary detail to demonstrate the population consequences of different sets of interventions targeted at different stages of the disease process. It can also accurately represent the effects of underlying changes in population structure and the concomitant competing effect of other major public health problems in specific groups (e.g., even without HIV infection the life expectancy of IV drug users will be much lower than in the general population—Vaillant, 1966).

In order to adequately represent the effects of the AIDS epidemic on health service use, one will also have to develop a set of service use models specific to demographic group and health characteristics. For example, the effects of prevention through education are most appropriately addressed at the noninfected population level, while combined chemotherapy is most useful for those with formal AIDS. The role of long-term care services is also probably best directed at those with formal AIDS. The amount and types of health services required are clearly driven by the demographic and health status model components, but, as more effective treatments and interventions are developed, feedback to the transition rates between health states will have to be modeled.

This model is also useful in strategic planning for data collection. That is, instead of generic data collection strategies that are likely to fail, the model could help identify the specific types of information that are required from very specific subpopulations at risk. By decomposing the data collection effort into a series of related small targeted efforts, one eliminates the management problems of very large field efforts and utilizes existing data from select populations and studies in a much more efficient fashion.

Models of Viral Behavior

The above models are designed to yield aggregate population estimates that are biologically realistic at the level of the individual human organism. These models do not, however, describe more elemental processes like the genetic drift of the virus, the co-factors that affect the latency of the virus or the direct effects of host characteristics on the natural history of the disease process. A different type of model is required to model these effects along with different types of data. For example, clinical data on antibody levels as a function of latency could be the basis for modeling the efficacy of treatment. Models of viral reservoirs (like the brain) could be used to examine the effect of drugs that cross the blood–brain barrier (e.g., peptide T, amantadine) and have their primary effect in the CNS. Models of such clinical efficacy and the effect of the physiological characteristics of the host in the disease process will help us to more precisely examine the effects of proposed interventions that, once modeled adequately, could be included in the population forecasting models. For example, if new chemotherapeutic protocols allow the long-term control of HIV infection, one will need to investigate what the health consequences are of the long-term latent infection (Edelson, 1988). Diabetes can be "controlled" in its acute manifestation, but we are just beginning to develop drug protocols to manage certain of its long-term morbid complications (e.g., atherosclerotic degeneration and collagen deposition in cardiac tissue due to impaired glucose metabolism). We do not currently know what the long-term effects of such management will be or if those strategies will continue to be effective for the immunologically less competent elderly person, thereby postponing the expression of HIV infection to advanced ages.

There are numerous examples of such models being used in the modeling of the effects of chronic disease processes on the U.S. population. The structure of the models to be employed may be of different types depending on the amount of information available on the physiological status of affected individuals. If information is limited, detailed compartment model strategies may be employed. These models have been successfully used to analyze the metabolism of drugs through a series of detailed metabolic stages in pharmacokinetic studies (e.g., Jacques, 1972). In those studies certain laboratory results may provide values (or ranges) of rate constants for certain states. Likewise one could view the virus operating in different organ systems or tissues as discrete compartments. Techniques for such nonlinear compartment models for neoplastic processes (involving incidence, growth, and treatment) are discussed in Manton and Stallard (1989).

Alternately, if measures are made on a number of variables describing the physiological state of an organism, certain general multivariate stochastic process models might be employed (e.g., Woodbury & Manton, 1983). A combination of both the stochastic compartment and process models is discussed in Yashin et al. (1988), as well as different likelihood estimation strategies.

Models of Long-Term Changes in the Disease and Its Impact

The type of detailed biological model described above had the intent of examining the effects of the virus in its current form on individual physiology. Given that long-term effects do not have to be represented in that model, certain simplifying assumptions could be employed. We now describe a third type of model for forecasting the evolution of the disease—toward our goal of anticipating potential changes in the characteristics of the epidemic. We know, for example, that the AIDS virus mutates rapidly (according to some estimates, about five times as fast as the influenza virus). This is one reason for the pessimism about the prospects for the development of an effective AIDS vaccine. This will certainly have implications for the type of vaccine to be developed (i.e., vaccines with different modes of action will have different likelihoods of being made obsolete by the genetic drift of the virus). Another type of long-term effect we will wish to model is the behavior of latent AIDS infection in the elderly where the immune system decreases in efficiency in certain ways. Does this mean that AIDS would necessarily be activated by age-related declines in the immune function? Would long-dormant AIDS become manifest as initiators in other types of neoplastic or autoimmune disorders at later ages if the individual managed to survive the direct effects of the AIDS virus? Will the disease expression of AIDS be quite different in persons where AIDS per se is controlled by, say, long-term AZT therapy? As more of the 1.5 million persons infected with the HIV virus reach long term, will they become more infectious and somehow trigger or rekindle the rate of incidence of the disease? And, in quite another vein, how will older people's attitudes and sexual behaviors enter in? All of these are long-term questions that must be anticipated if we are not simply to be reacting, belatedly, to innovations in the disease process and to changes in public awareness and behaviors.

The structure of models used to evaluate such changes will be somewhat different than in the population forecasting case in that more data on individual physiology and behavior will be needed in the models. Thus these models will be more like multivariate stochastic process models (Manton & Stallard, 1988; Woodbury & Manton, 1983), except that exogenous changes must be introduced into them. These exogenous forces represent the socioenvironmental factors inducing viral changes that emerge over the long term (e.g., Yashin et al., 1989a).

AGENDA FOR RESEARCH

We view the development of appropriate, biosocially realistic forecasting and monitoring models as the most important research agenda for detecting early manifestations of the AIDS epidemic and anticipating the emergent impact on the elderly. The development of such sophisticated modeling and forecasting cannot be achieved through a casual effort; it requires the resolution of basic statistical problems and the manipulation and analysis of large amounts of quite heterogeneous data. Moreover, efforts to develop such models must begin now because there will be a considerable lag period between the initial efforts at modeling and the emergence of satisfactory models. Such a lag is not only important for model development but also essential for the development and testing of vaccines and clinical treatments. Concomitant with this modeling effort is the need to conduct special, highly targeted data collection efforts to fill in the knowledge gaps that are identified in the forecasting models.

That forecasting models of the kind we advocate can be successful in anticipating—and reacting early to—changes in public health is, ironically, currently being evidenced in the area of chronic disease prevention in developing countries. Currently, the demographic structures of many developing countries make the overall impact of chronic disease small. However, with the success of population control programs and the rise in life expectancy in many developing countries, the increase in the public health importance of chronic diseases can be predicted with a high (near certain) degree of confidence. As a consequence, adverse changes in health behavior in those countries will be amplified by basic demographic shifts. That appropriate forecasting models can influence policy makers was demonstrated at a meeting of health ministers from 35 countries at the World Health Organization World Health Assembly in Geneva. These ministers found entirely credible the forecasts from a biosocially sophisticated program (Manton & Dowd, 1988), although they had rejected the results from less sophisticated models as not scientifically valid. As a consequence, action was initiated on smoking reduction campaigns in several countries (despite short-term tax revenue incentives to the contrary).

In addition to their potential success in influencing policy, a further motivation for such forecasting activities is that they represent true advances in the scientific understanding of a type of epidemic that we are just beginning to recognize. Thus development of such tools constitutes an investment in the advancement of basic scientific understanding of fundamental health processes (e.g., the relation of chronic viral infection and viral drift to chronic disease manifestations and aging). Such understandings, with their major consequences for the nation's elderly, have to date received relatively little attention. Thus further development and use of sophisticated forecasting procedures may help to sensitize us to a broader range of other similar deleterious health processes impacting the elderly, such as those that are driven by the interaction of slow viruses and autoimmune response.

In sum, as we stated at the outset, appropriate models are needed to meet a variety of goals: for example, for observing possible changes in the disease process in specific subpopulations of older people; for estimating the effects of the epidemic on survival, and on older people's future needs for health care; and for evaluating interventions both in disease prevention and in methods of treatment. Without appropriate modeling, professional and policy programs may well neglect the special vulnerability of older people—physiological, social, and economic. Older adults, who are physiologically vulnerable because of the lowering of immunocompetency with age, are also economically vulnerable because of their high per capita consumption of acute and long-term care services; thus it is older people who are especially likely to be caught in the competition with AIDS victims for scarce health services. As a major agenda item, improved forecasting can become a critically important guide in meeting such goals.

APPENDIX

We present a formal representation of an area-specific seroprevalence rate in terms of rates estimated from STD clinic surveillance, a homosexual survey, probabilities of self-selection into STD clinics and/or compliance for seropositivity testing in a survey, and prevalence rates of gay men and/or STD-infected individuals in the overall population. These are the ingredients necessary to construct seroprevalence rates when random sampling is not feasible and estimates must be produced from multiple convenience samples.

Let

$$X = \begin{cases} 1 \text{ if an individual is HIV-positive} \\ 0 \text{ otherwise} \end{cases}$$

$$S_1 = \begin{cases} 1 \text{ if an individual has an STD} \\ 0 \text{ otherwise} \end{cases}$$

$$S_2 = \begin{cases} 1 \text{ if an individual voluntarily self-selects to visit an STD clinic and} \\ \quad \text{be tested for seropositivity} \\ 0 \text{ otherwise} \end{cases}$$

$$H_1 = \begin{cases} 1 \text{ if an individual is a homosexual} \\ 0 \text{ otherwise} \end{cases}$$

$$H_2 = \begin{cases} 1 \text{ if a homosexual individual is surveyed and agrees to seropositivity testing} \\ 0 \text{ otherwise} \end{cases}$$

We want to calculate $\text{Prob}(X=1)$, which we will interpret as an overall seroprevalence rate, in terms of ascertainable rates from self-selected subpopulations and selection probabilities. To this end, we repeatedly apply the definition of conditional probability to obtain the representation

$$\begin{aligned} \text{Prob}(X=1) = {} & \text{Prob}(X=1 \mid H_2=1, H_1=1)\ \text{Prob}(H_2=1 \mid H_1=1)\ \text{Prob}(H_1=1) \\ & + \text{Prob}(X=1 \mid H_2=0, H_1=1)\ \text{Prob}(H_2=0 \mid H_1=1)\ \text{Prob}(H_1=1) \\ & + \text{Prob}(X=1, H_2=0, H_1=0) \end{aligned} \quad (1)$$

In the first term, $\text{Prob}(X=1 \mid H_2=1, H_1=1)$ is estimated from the survey of homosexuals and stabilized via Empirical Bayes strategies using data on homosexuals from regions other than the one currently being assessed. The quantity $\text{Prob}(H_2=1 \mid H_1=1)$ is interpreted as the fraction of the homosexual population surveyed *and* agreeing to seropositivity testing. $\text{Prob}(H_1=1)$ is the proportion of the regional population estimated to be homosexuals. The first component of the second term in the above expansion is further decomposed as

$$\begin{aligned} & \text{Prob}(X=1 \mid H_2=0, H_1=1) \\ & = [\text{Prob}(X=1 \mid S_1=1, S_2=1, H_2=0, H_1=1)\ \text{Prob}(S_2=1 \mid S_1=1, H_2=0, H_1=1) \\ & \quad + \text{Prob}(X=1 \mid S_1=1, S_2=0, H_2=0, H_1=1)\ \text{Prob}(S_2=0 \mid S_1=1, H_2=0, H_1=1)] \\ & \quad + \text{Prob}(S_1=1 \mid H_2=0, H_1=1) \end{aligned} \quad (2)$$

The conditional probability $\text{Prob}(X=1 \mid S_1=1, S_2=1, H_2=0, H_1=1)$ is estimable from STD clinic data; however, $\text{Prob}(X=1 \mid S_1=1, S_2=0, H_2=0, H_1=1)$ must be inferred indirectly, possibly from gonorrhea prevalence rates (see, in this regard, Pickering et al., 1986).

The third term also requires further decomposition as

$$\begin{aligned} & [\text{Prob}(X=1 \mid S_2=1, S_1=1, H_1=0)\ \text{Prob}(S_2=1 \mid S_1=1, H_1=0) \\ & \quad + \text{Prob}(X=1 \mid S_2=0, S_1=1, H_1=0)\ \text{Prob}(S_2=0 \mid S_1=1, H_1=0] \\ & \quad \times \text{Prob}(S_1=1 \mid H_1=0) \times \text{Prob}(H_1=0) \end{aligned}$$

The conditional probability $\text{Prob}(X = 1 \mid S_2 = 1, S_1 = 1, H_1 = 0)$ is estimable from STD clinic volunteers, while $\text{Prob}(X = 1 \mid S_2 = 0, S_1 = 1, H_1 = 0)$ requires indirect estimation, again possible utilizing rates for gonorrhea. All components of these decompositions must either be directly estimated or judgmentally assumed (based on some substantive rationale, however coarse) in order to estimate $\text{Prob}(X = 1)$ for a given geographic region. A much more elaborate version—involving more than two kinds of population data—of this program is in serious need of implementation in the United States, Western Europe, and Africa.

REFERENCES

Anderson, R.M., G.C. Medley, R.M. May, and A.N. Johnson. 1986. "A Preliminary Study of the Transmission Dynamics of the Human Immunodeficiency Virus (HIV), the Causal Agent of AIDS." *Institute of Mathematics Journal of Mathematics Applied in Medicine and Biology* 3:229–263.

Berkman, L., B. Singer, and K.G. Manton. 1989. "Black/White Differences in Health Status and Mortality among the Elderly." *Demography* (in press).

Bongaarts, J. 1987. *A Model of the Spread of HIV Infection and the Demographic Impact of AIDS.* Presented at IOM Workshop on Mathematical Modeling of the Spread of Human Immunodeficiency Virus and the Demographic Impact of AIDS, Washington, DC, October 15–17.

Brookmeyer, R., and G. Mitchell. 1986. "The Minimum Size of the AIDS Epidemic in the United States." *Lancet* 2:1320–1322.

Centers for Disease Control. 1987. "Human Immunodeficiency Virus Infection in the United States: A Review of Current Knowledge." CDC Report, Nov. 30, 1987, prepared by J.J. Dondero et al.

Curran, J.W., H.W. Jaffe, A.M. Hardy, W.M. Morgan, R.M. Selik, and T. Dondero. 1988. "Epidemiology of HIV Infection and AIDS in the United States." *Science* 239:610–616.

Dietz, K. 1988. "The Dynamics of Spread of HIV in the Heterosexual Population." Pp.77–105 in *Statistical Analysis and Mathematical Modeling of AIDS,* edited by J.C. Jager and E. Euitenberg. Oxford, England: Oxford University Press.

Edelson, R.L. 1988. "Light-Activated Drugs." *Scientific American* 259:68–75.

Fischl, M.A., D.D. Richman, M.H. Greico, M.S. Gottleib, P.A. Volberding, O.L. Laskin, J.M. Leedon, J.E. Groopman, D. Mildvan, R.T. Schooly, G.G. Jackson, D.T. Durack, D. King, and AZT Collaborative Working Group. 1987. "The Efficacy of Azidothymidine (AZT) in the Treatment of Patients with AIDS and AIDS-Related Complex: A Double-Blind, Placebo-Controlled Trial." *New England Journal of Medicine* 317:187–191.

Halloran, M.E., and C.J. Struchiner. 1988. "Prevention of AIDS in Intravenous Drug Users and Its Consequences on the Epidemic in an Interacting Heterosexual Population." Draft manuscript, Department of Population Sciences, Harvard School of Public Health.

Haywood, A.M. 1986. "Patterns of Persistent Viral Infections." *New England Journal of Medicine* 315:939–948.
Hethcote, H.W., and J.A. Yorke. 1983. *Gonorrhea Transmission Dynamics and Control: Lecture Notes on Biomathematics.* New York: Springer-Verlag.
Ho, D., R.J. Pomerantz, and J.C. Kaplan. 1987. "Pathogenesis of Infection with Human Immunodeficiency Virus." *New England Journal of Medicine* 317:278–286.
Hughes, W.T. 1987. "Pneumocystis Carinii Pneumonitis." *New England Journal of Medicine* 317:1021–1023.
Jacques, J.A. 1972. *Compartmental Analysis in Biology and Medicine.* Amsterdam: Elsevier.
Katzman, R. 1986. "Alzheimer's Disease." *New England Journal of Medicine* 314:964–973.
Lambert, B. 1988. "AIDS Count: Is the Quest for Precision on the Right Track?" *New York Times* July 24.
Manton, K.G. 1987. "Forecasting Health Status Changes in an Aging U.S. Population: Assessment of the Current Status and Some Proposals." *Climatic Change* 11:179–210.
Manton, K.G., and J.E. Dowd. 1988. *Demonstration of Chronic Disease Forecasting Model.* Paper presented at the World Health Assembly, Geneva, Switzerland, World Health Organization, May.
Manton, K.G., and E. Stallard. 1989. *Chronic Disease Modeling.* London: Charles Griffin.
Manton, K.G., E. Stallard, M.A. Woodbury, W.B. Riggan, J.P. Creason, and T.J. Mason. 1987. "Statistically Adjusted Estimates of Geographic Mortality Profiles." *Journal of the National Cancer Institute* 78:805–815.
Manton, K.G., M.A. Woodbury, E. Stallard, W.B. Riggan, J.P. Creasan, and A.C. Pellom. 1989 (in press). "Empirical Bayes Procedures for Stabilizing Maps of U.S. Cancer Mortality Rates." *Journal of the American Statistical Association.*
May, R.M., and R.M. Anderson. 1987. "Transmission Dynamics of HIV Infection." *Nature* 328:719–721.
Morgan, W.M., and J.W. Curran. 1986. "Acquired Immune Deficiency Syndrome: Current and Future Trends." *Public Health Reports* 101:459–464.
Pickering, J., J. Wiley, N.S. Padian, L.E. Lieb, D.F. Echenberg, and J. Walker. 1986. "Modeling the Incidence of Acquired Immunodeficiency Syndrome (AIDS) in San Francisco, Los Angeles, and New York." *Mathematical Modeling* 7:661–688.
Riggan, W.B., J.P. Creason, W.C. Nelson, K.G. Manton, E. Stallard, M.A. Woodbury, A.C. Pellom, and J. Beaubier. 1987. *U.S. Cancer Mortality Rate and Trends, 1950–1979. Volume IV: Maps.* United States Environmental Protection Agency Health Effects Research Laboratory, EPA/600/1-83/105d. Washington, DC: U.S. Government Printing Office.
Rothenberg, R., M. Woelfel, R. Stoneburner, J. Milberg, R. Parker, and B. Truman. 1987. "Survival with the Acquired Immunodeficiency Syndrome: Experience with 5833 Cases in New York City." *New England Journal of Medicine* 317:1297–1302.
Vaillant, G.E. 1966. "A 12-Year Follow Up of New York Narcotic Addicts: II The Natural History of a Chronic Disease." *New England Journal of Medicine* 275:1282–1288.
Weinberg, D.S., and H.W. Murray. 1987. "Coping with AIDS: The Special Problems of New York City." *New England Journal of Medicine* 317:1469–1473.
Woodbury, M.A., and K.G. Manton. 1983. "A Theoretical Model of the Physiological Dynamics of Circulatory Diseases. *Human Biology* 55:417–441.

Yashin, A.I., K.G. Manton, and E. Stallard. 1989. "The Propagation of Uncertainty in Human Mortality Processes Operating in Stochastic Environments." *Theoretical Population Biology* forthcoming.

Yashin, A.I., K.G. Manton, and E. Stallard. 1989a. "The Propagation of Uncertainty in Human Mortality Processes Operating in Stochastic Environments." In review at *Theoretical Population Biology.*

Yashin, A.I., K.G. Manton, and E. Stallard. 1989b. "Active Life Expectancy Stochastic Process Models." Center for Demographic Studies, Duke University, Durham, North Carolina.

CHAPTER 10

The Social Consequences of the AIDS Epidemic: A Challenge for the Social Sciences

Yasmine Ergas

Responding to the challenge that AIDS presents, the Social Science Research Council, drawing on formulations of the problems raised by AIDS that were proposed in several Council meetings, has been developing a research agenda centered on the epidemic's projected social consequences. The agenda aims to inform society's coping strategies and, if possible, to forestall negative effects while encouraging the positive innovations to which health crises sometimes give rise. The importance of turning the attention of the social sciences to the social effects of the disease is becoming more evident every day.[1] This article attempts to set a framework for studying the social consequences of the epidemic by highlighting the kinds of problems on which research and theoretical work must focus. It does not presume to prescribe the content of appropriate research or social theory.

Adapted, with permission from the Social Science Research Council (605 Third Avenue, New York, N.Y. 10058), from the article under this title published by the Council in *Items*, Vol. 41, Nos. 3/4, December 1987, pp. 33–39.

Yasmine Ergas, a sociologist, is a staff associate at the Social Science Research Council, New York. During 1987-88, she was on leave at the Institute for Advanced Study (Princeton, New Jersey). Richard A. Berk has been the leading proponant of an approach focusing on the special consequences of the HIV/AIDS epidemic, and much of this article is indebted to him. It has also benefited from the contributions of those who have attended Council planning meetings and of other Council staff members, in particular Richard C. Rockwell and David L. Sills.

[1] Before examining some of these effects in greater detail, a caveat is in order. AIDS—Acquired Immune Deficiency Syndrome—has come to denote, both in casual conversation and, to a significant degree, in scientific discussion, HIV infection in general. As medical researchers have shown, infection with HIV proceeds on a continuum, although progression from one state to the next is not automatic. Many individuals, in the United States and elsewhere, are and may remain at the first stage of this infection. It is now expected, however, that a significantly large proportion of those infected will develop AIDS-related symptoms and that many others will go on to suffer from AIDS.

All forms of HIV infection raise pressing policy issues, ranging from the promotion of public health to the protection of civil liberties, from the provision of medical and social services to the coordination of internationally sanctioned measures. Furthermore, they all possess the potential to provoke significant social and cultural change. It is with this broad range of issues—and with the implications of different stages and manifestations of infection and illness—that we need to be and, indeed, are concerned.

THE SOCIAL CONSEQUENCES OF AIDS: AN OVERVIEW

Historically, epidemics have both shaped and been shaped by the structures of social, economic, and political life. Their course has been affected by behavioral patterns, popular beliefs, health care services, and governmental responses. And their demographic, economic, legislative, and cultural effects have often outlived the diseases that created them. Smallpox, cholera, tuberculosis, polio, and the bubonic plague are, in a sense, still with us even though, in the Western world, the numbers of the stricken have been drastically reduced.

The legacies of disease inform the knowledge on which a significant amount of medical science, as well as many constitutive features of contemporary societies, now rests. From the immunizations routinely performed to the power of public health authorities, from common understandings of "purity and danger" to shared assumptions regarding health and illness, from the ethics of the healing professions and the organization of medical care to the regulation of immigration, the great epidemics of the past structure our experiences of the present.[2]

In this legacy, the accumulation of scientific knowledge plays a special role. Such knowledge as has been possessed has generally been mobilized to cope with disease. In turn, this knowledge has been profoundly affected by the issues that diseases have placed on the scientific agenda.

From both a societal and a scientific perspective, AIDS promises to be no different. Exacting a significant toll in terms of human lives, threatening a virtual decimation of populations that engage in "high-risk behaviors," the current epidemic is already meting out tragedy and engendering social change. It is also prompting new public and private policies and generating scientific breakthroughs. Until now, the mobilization of science seems to have especially

[2] The phrase "purity and danger" is borrowed from Douglas (1966). On epidemics, their "social construction," and their historical effects, see Brandt (1987), Carmichael (1986), McNeill (1976), and Rosenberg (1962).

involved biomedical and epidemiological researchers, while the potential contributions of the social sciences—and the significance for them of confronting the questions the current epidemic raises—appear to have received relatively scanty and generally fragmentary attention.

Need for Social Science Research

Yet the social implications of AIDS—its epidemiological dependence on particular patterns of social behavior and its potential impact on the organization of social life—have been recognized as being of paramount importance. The transmission of AIDS takes place through specific behavioral routes, including (among others) sexual, parenteral, and perinatal contact. Acknowledging that "neither vaccines nor satisfactory drug therapies for HIV or AIDS are likely to be available in the near future," the National Academy of Sciences and the Institute of Medicine urged as early as 1986 that a series of social measures be taken to curb the spread of the epidemic and to deal with its effects. Referring explicitly to the potential contributions of the social sciences, the National Academy and the Institute of Medicine report stressed:

> Social science research can help develop effective education programs . . . (that) contribute to the design of policies that reduce the public's fear of AIDS and that help eliminate discriminatory practices toward AIDS patients. And it can shape the establishment of health care and social services for AIDS patients. (Institute of Medicine, 1986, p. 27)

This is but an initial suggestion of the ways in which the social sciences can contribute to the development of coping strategies. As the Academy report suggests, the task before the social sciences is urgent and exacting. It requires marshalling expertise that is presently scattered across a multiplicity of disciplines; it requires developing a dialogue capable of extending beyond the borders of the social sciences to engage policy makers, epidemiologists, and biomedical researchers; and it requires assessing the changes that the current epidemic has already set in motion and those that it is likely to produce.

The effects of AIDS determine the context within which the efforts of the social sciences must be situated and provide important data on which to base further research. Viewed in an international perspective, AIDS threatens entire societies. In some parts of Africa, for instance, where the disease affects both sexes in approximately equal numbers, the effects of AIDS are already widespread. But even in countries where the epidemic has been characterized by a "Western" epidemiological pattern—largely confined initially to male homosexuals, intravenous drug abusers, and their sexual partners and children—the consequences of AIDS are significant.

In the United States, these effects are beginning to be discernible in the cultural and behavioral patterns of specific social groups and in the institutions that bind society together. Culturally, AIDS has called renewed attention to sex and sexuality, awakened fears of contagion and epidemic disasters, and inspired a new literature of disease. The mass media provide almost daily coverage of the AIDS epidemic, often stressing the implications of the disease for sexual practices and mores. Such coverage has the collateral effect of giving both sex and sexuality greater salience in public discourse. Institutionally, AIDS has become a factor influencing international as well as domestic policy and politics.

Social Cleavages

Both culturally and institutionally, the epidemic has highlighted existing fault lines in American society while provoking new tensions and prompting new choices. It has, for instance, reinforced the stigma and discrimination experienced by those groups among whom the disease has been especially virulent: male homosexuals and intravenous drug abusers.[3] And since inner-city minorities are disproportionately represented among AIDS sufferers, the epidemic has also given renewed salience to the racial cleavages that divide American society, for AIDS occurs far more frequently among black and Hispanic men, women, and children than it does among whites.

While AIDS is posing an especially serious threat to populations that have historically been severely disadvantaged, it has also raised new questions that both polarize and reorder societal priorities and beliefs. Should sexuality that deviates from the canonical model of heterosexual matrimonial monogamy be publicly acknowledged and perhaps implicitly condoned? Proponents of differing views form opposing camps, while new alliances are forged between traditional "liberals"—like Representative Waxman—and equally traditional "conservatives"—like Surgeon General C. Everett Koop.

Alterations in Everyday Affairs

As debates touching upon themes such as these unfold, catalyzing widespread public attention, AIDS alters the features of everyday life—and death—for those populations that are most dramatically affected. In New York and San Francisco, among the minorities that live in the inner cities, but also in the art world and the design industry, AIDS is a daily experience—of loss, fear, stigmatization, destitution, and discrimination; and, too rarely, solidarity and community support.

[3] On the psychological and social stresses associated with AIDS, with particular reference to homosexual men, see Emmons et al. (1986), Joseph et al. (1984; 1987; n.d.), and Kessler et al. (n.d.).

At the same time, AIDS has appeared on the agenda of the major institutions of American society, affecting the ways in which services are provided and governance is ensured. AIDS has become an issue for private enterprise as well as for national and local government, for the health system and the insurance industry, for the educational system and the courts, for the armed forces and the foreign service.

Within each institutional arena, the epidemic elicits policy responses, often provoking changes that have extensive ramifications. These policies sometimes take the findings of the social sciences into account. More often, they evolve in a piecemeal manner, and, because data regarding their characteristics and effects are not systematically gathered, they yield little information that may be of use in future decision making.

Problems of Influencing Behavior

Foremost on the public agenda is the issue of effective education. Health officials, private enterprise, and agencies of the federal government are engaged in a myriad of activities designed to promote awareness and behavioral change while forestalling panic. These initiatives are rarely monitored for their ability to achieve their aims, yet the belief that information—or education—suffices to affect behavior in the intended direction is seriously open to question. As a basis for effective education, research must probe more deeply into the effects of fear, and into risk taking, and beliefs about health. Even more importantly, the factors that lead from knowledge to awareness and action must be garnered, as the extensive social science literature on mass communication and mass persuasion is relevant to AIDS. If it is imperative that neither the public nor policy makers succumb to illusions regarding the import of information, it is equally important to understand which campaigns have succeeded and when, how, why, and which are likely to do so in the future.

Implications for Health Care Facilities

At the same time as the question of education is being broached, public health officials and hospital administrators are developing strategies designed to meet the multiple demands AIDS places on medical facilities. AIDS generates pressures for beds, trained professional staff, and adequately prepared volunteer personnel (cf. Institute of Medicine 1986, pp. 150–157). Public health officials and administrators must decide whether AIDS sufferers should be placed in "dedicated" (that is, segregated) wards or integrated with other patients. They must also deal with the growing demand AIDS produces for mental health services and with the type of counseling this epidemic requires, for AIDS entails coping with both loss and danger—a situation that can create complex anxiety and depression reactions that are particularly difficult to treat.

Economic Burdens

Public health officials, hospital administrators, and the society as a whole must confront the economic burden that AIDS imposes. Estimates of the average lifetime costs of the care required by an AIDS sufferer, from diagnosis to death, range from $27,600 to $150,000 (as estimated back in 1986), with the total costs of care estimated at between $8 billion and $16 billion by 1991.[4] The direct costs of this disease are partially financed by insurance companies. But AIDS sufferers are frequently required to pay for a significant portion of their care and they often cannot do so. AIDS generally impairs the ability to maintain employment, thus imposing severe financial hardship on the ill and a general loss of productivity on the economy. And since for many the loss of employment spells the loss of health insurance, Medicaid and local government revenues must cover the unreimbursed costs of medical care for AIDS sufferers. The epidemic has therefore contributed both to stimulating the search for new solutions to the financing of health care and to renewed debates over the adequacy of present arrangements.

POLICY DEBATES

These debates have led in two directions: on the one hand, insurers have pressed for the right to test insurance applicants for HIV seropositivity; on the other, critics of the current system have called attention to the responsibility of public institutions for ensuring adequate health care for the entire population (see Fox, 1986; Hammond & Shapiro, 1986, pp. 143–167; Oppenheimer & Padgug, 1986). The discussions that have developed on the issue of health care financing may foreshadow changes that would dovetail with other transformative processes that AIDS appears to have already set in motion.

When the AIDS epidemic began, historians have noted, the health polity was in a state of flux, shifting attention from infectious diseases to chronic degenerative diseases; from the promise of science to its unrealized potential; from comprehensive service provisions to cost control.[5] At a minimum, AIDS has redirected attention to infectious diseases and, therefore, to the public health

[4] Variations in estimates reflect differences in the methodologies employed as well as in the medical sites examined. The costs of care also appear to vary in relation to the particular symptomatology of the AIDS case (patients with *pneumocystis carinii* appear to incur higher costs than those with Kaposzi's sarcoma) and the social characteristics of the patient. On the costs of health care for AIDS sufferers, see Institute of Medicine (1986, pp. 155–175), and Scitovsky & Cline (1986).

[5] The term "health polity" is used in the sense defined in Fox (1986), page 7, to mean "the ways a community . . . conceives of and organizes its response to health and illness." The description of the transformations the health polity is undergoing is also derived from this article by Fox. See also Starr (1982).

measures that such diseases require. It is prompting a critical reexamination of existing legislative and administrative measures, such as those regarding communicable and sexually transmitted diseases (Gostin, 1986; Kuller & Kingsley, 1986; Musto, 1986).

Public Health and Individual Liberties

At a more general level, AIDS is stimulating a far-reaching discussion over the relationship between public health and individual liberties, with significant implications for the relationship between the state (understood in its broadest sense) and civil society.[6] The exercise of compulsory public health powers for the good of the community involves a potentially massive infringement of individual liberty, autonomy, and privacy. Yet public health jurisprudence has been a relatively neglected area of the law. Addressing the classic question for public health jurisprudence—to what extent may the state require its citizens to submit to restraint or loss of rights in order to interrupt the spread of disease?—many have expressed the fear that AIDS may occasion new, and coercive, measures for the "policing of society." Others have emphasized the attention that public health officials and legislatures have thus far given to individual rights. In this context, scholars and activists have drawn attention to the ways in which public health measures relating to venereal disease have been used to control prostitution. "Quarantine," writes Musto (1986, p. 108), "is a response not only to the actual mode of transmission, but also to a popular demand to establish a boundary between the kind of person so diseased and the respectable people who hope to remain healthy." (Also see Gostin, 1986, especially pp. 87–88, and Brandt, 1987.)

Mobilization of Support Groups

Concomitantly, the ways in which the demand for services for AIDS sufferers are being addressed, and the importance attributed to solidary organizations and to the mobilization of voluntary groups, are placing the necessity for complementing and sustaining such service-providing groups on the public agenda. By 1986 the establishment and consolidation of advocacy organizations concerned with the ways in which the epidemic was being confronted had already added to the panoply of preexisting interests, social movement organizations, and voluntary associations a new set of actors whose influence

[6] Out of a rapidly developing literature on the issue of the relationship between civil liberties and public health as these pertain to the AIDS epidemic, see Relman et al. (1985), Levine et al. (1986), Bayer, Levine, and Wolf (1986), and Bayer (1986). On the effects of quarantine, see Musto (1986). As an example of the social mobilization that can be generated by public health regulations, see Walkowitz (1980).

may well continue to be felt even after the epidemic is halted. Among these organizations are the American Foundation for AIDS Research (AMFAR), the Gay Men's Health Crisis of New York, and the National AIDS Network.

But the organizations that developed early in the wake of the AIDS epidemic may not correspond to the needs of all populations. The inner-city minorities among whom the epidemic is attaining particular virulence, for instance, may be underserviced by organizations whose original impetus came from within other communities. Social scientists concerned with the organization of American politics, the role of social movements, and the importance of the voluntary sector in the provision of social services can offer useful suggestions on the ways in which the AIDS organizations can be supported. For example, Sills (1957) has shown how voluntary associations can outlive their original purposes and yet consolidate their organization by developing new goals, and others have described the far-reaching impact of social movements associated with health (see Nissenbaum, 1980; Levitt & Numbers, 1985; and Rosenberg, 1962, especially pp. 213–225).

Accentuation of Civil Rights Issues

Policy issues are also raised as existing differentiations in the distribution of civil liberties and social rights become accentuated. Branches of the federal government, for instance, have initiated systematic screening of their personnel. In 1985, the Department of Defense began testing all applicants for entry into the military services. Screening was then extended to all active duty personnel Screening has led to a reduction in the population of possible recruits. At a time when seropositivity among applicants nationally averaged 1.6 per 1,000, the military services were finding that up to 20 per 1,000 recruit applicants from high-incidence areas were seropositive (Institute of Medicine, 1986, p. 68). Screening may also affect posting decisions, for the military services stationed overseas have been perceived as transmitters of the disease. Thus, allegations that the American armed forces have spread AIDS to the local population have entered into discussions regarding the renewal of the American bases in the Philippines and have provoked angry polemics in Japan. Concern with considerations linked to international relations has also led the Foreign Service to screen its personnel. In December 1986, the State Department announced that a test for HIV seropositivity would be required of all its employees and their dependents over the age of 18 who are stationed overseas. Seropositive employees—or employees with seropositive dependents—would be restricted to certain posts so as to prevent potential damage to foreign relations. And, as with the armed forces, testing in the Foreign Service may have repercussions on recruitment pools as well as on the character of the relations that develop between seronegative and seropositive individuals.

SUMMARY

The current epidemic calls, then, for critical choices and has the potential for provoking significant changes. From the military to the schools, from prisons to hospitals, from civil rights and the enforcement of laws to the employment relationship, from sexual mores and even the understanding of sexuality to the ability of people to travel freely both across and within national boundaries, AIDS has exerted or may soon exert a powerful influence. It can also promote innovation, as society comes to grips with the challenge this dreadful disease poses. It has led to the formation of new organizational structures and to new solidarities. It may yet lead to new definitions of rights and obligations, to new understandings of death and dying, and to new rituals for coping with disease (cf. Musto, 1986, p. 115). It has led, and will in all likelihood continue to lead, to new scientific research and discoveries in the social as well as the biomedical sciences, as in the studies of sexual behavior, IV drug abuse, and the impact of the AIDS epidemic on historical understandings of disease (Rosenberg, 1986). Ultimately the effects of AIDS will reflect society's ability to marshal the knowledge at its disposal and to generate new types and sources of knowledge in order to limit the spread and the damage of disease.

The task before the social sciences is complex. It requires understanding to what extent and how this epidemic will (1) affect the structures of everyday life, (2) reorder social groupings, (3) harden boundaries, (4) redefine gender and sex roles, (5) affect life cycles and family cycles, and (6) exert an impact on basic social institutions, from the health care system to the labor market. Without succumbing to the illusory appeal of social engineering, and aware of the unintended consequences of social action, one is prompted to ask: What can be done not only to curtail this epidemic but also to cope with its effects? The Social Science Research Council's agenda seeks to provide answers to this question.

REFERENCES

Bayer, Ronald. 1986. "AIDS, Power and Reason." *The Milbank Quarterly* 64:168–182, Supplement I.

Bayer, Ronald, Carol Levine, and Susan M. Wolf. 1986. "HIV Antibody Screening: A Ethical Framework to Evaluate Proposed Programs." *Journal of the American Medical Association* 256–613:1768–1774.

Brandt, Alan M. 1987. *No Magic Bullet: A Social History of Venereal Disease in the United States Since 1880.* New York: Oxford University Press.

Carmichael, Ann G. 1986. *Plague and the Poor in Renaissance Florence.* Cambridge, U.K.: Cambridge University Press.

Emmons, Carol-Ann et al. 1986. "Psychosocial Predictors of Reported Behavior Change in Homosexual Men at Risk for AIDS." *Health Education Quarterly* 13(4):331–345.

Fox, Daniel M. 1986. "AIDS and the American Health Polity: The History and Prospects of a Crisis of Authority." *The Milbank Quarterly* 64:7–33, Supplement I.

Gostin, Larry. 1986. "The Future of Communicable Disease Control: Toward a New Concept in Public Health Law." *The Milbank Quarterly* 64:79–96, Supplement I.

Hammond, J.D., and Arnold F. Shapiro. 1986. "AIDS and the Limits of Insurability." *The Milbank Quarterly* 64:143–167, Supplement I.

Institute of Medicine, National Academy of Sciences. 1986. *Confronting AIDS: Directions for Public Health, Health Care and Research.* Washington, DC: National Academy Press.

Joseph, Jill G. et al. 1984. "Coping with the Threat of AIDS: An Approach to Psychosocial Assessment." *American Psychologist* 39:1297–1302.

Joseph, Jill G. et al. 1987. "Magnitude and Determinants of Behavioral Risk Reduction: Longitudinal Analysis of a Cohort at Risk for AIDS." *Psychology and Health.*

Joseph, Jill G. et al. n.d. "Perceived Risk of AIDS: Assessing the Behavioral and Psychosocial Consequences in a Cohort of Gay Men."

Kessler, Ronald C. et al. n.d. "Effects of HIV Infection: Perceived Health and Clinical Status on a Cohort at Risk for AIDS."

Kuller, Lewis H., and Lawrence A. Kingsley. 1986. "The Epidemic of AIDS: A Failure of Public Health Policy." *The Milbank Quarterly* 64:56–78, Supplement I.

Levine, Carol et al. 1986. "AIDS: Public Health and Civil Liberties." *Hastings Center Report, Special Supplement.*

Levitt, Judith Walzer, and Ronald L. Numbers, eds. 1985. *Sickness and Health in America: Readings in the History of Medicine and Public Health.* Madison: University of Wisconsin Press.

McNeill, William H. 1976. *Plagues and People.* Garden City, NY: Anchor Press.

Musto, David F. 1986. "Quarantine and the Problem of AIDS." *The Milbank Quarterly* 64:56–117, Supplement I.

Nissenbaum, Stephen. 1980. *Sex, Diet and Debility in Jacksonian America: Sylvester Graham and Health Reform.* Westport, CT: Greenwood Press.

Oppenheimer, Gerard M., and Robert A. Padgug. 1986. "AIDS: The Risks to Insurers, the Threat to Equity." *Hastings Center Report* 18–22.

Relman, Arnold S. et al. 1985. "AIDS: The Emerging Ethical Dilemmas." *Hastings Center Report, Special Supplement* 15–4.

Rosenberg, Charles E. 1962. *The Cholera Years: The United States in 1832, 1849, and 1866.* Chicago: University of Chicago Press.

———. 1986. "Disease and Social Order in America: Perceptions and Expectations." *The Milbank Quarterly* 64:34–55, Supplement I.

Scitovsky, Anne A., and M. Cline. 1986. "Medical Care Costs of Patients with AIDS in San Francisco." *Journal of the American Medical Association* 256:3107–3109.

Sills, David L. 1957. *The Volunteers: Means and Ends in a National Organization.* New York: Free Press.

Starr, Paul. 1982. *The Social Transformation of American Medicine.* New York: Basic Books.

Walkowitz, Judith R. 1980. *Prostitution and Victorian Society: Women, Class, and the State.* Cambridge, U.K.: Cambridge University Press.

CHAPTER 11

Notes for the Future: Research, Prevention, Care, Public Policy

Marcia G. Ory and Diane Zablotsky

The widespread neglect of older people as a target population for AIDS research, service, public education, and policy has been documented throughout this volume. We believe that this set of chapters presents, for the first time, a comprehensive picture of the magnitude of AIDS in the older population and the impact of the current and projected AIDS epidemic on older people—as persons with AIDS (PWA), as informal and formal caregivers of persons with AIDS, as competitors for limited health care dollars and personnel, and as citizens in a society whose social institutions have both shaped and been shaped by the AIDS epidemic.

These "Notes" are added at the end to provide a brief summary of what we need to know about the nature and consequences of AIDS today and to suggest some of the future problems and issues in an aging society. Like the individual chapters, these "Notes for the Future" will focus primarily on the social science research arena. However, health care, education, and policy issues that are also informed by scientific knowledge will not be ignored.

One of our underlying assumptions has been that the AIDS epidemic highlights gaps already existing in research and exacerbates longstanding problems in health care and society. It is our contention that a better understanding of the social and behavioral aspects of AIDS in the middle and later years will increase basic knowledge in many related areas (e.g., human sexuality, informal and formal caregiving arrangements, behavioral change techniques) and contribute to the improvement of health care models and policies for a wider array of illnesses and populations.

THE COMPLEXITY OF AIDS

The complex nature of AIDS has been emphasized throughout this volume. Until this recent epidemic, scientific attention and public health concern in Western nations was turning from infectious diseases to chronic degenerative diseases. AIDS refocuses our attention to issues of infectious diseases. Yet, unlike earlier infectious diseases, AIDS has both acute and chronic manifestations, requiring combinations of intensive medical treatment and long-term care over the course of the disease. Even after the development of AIDS, some persons experience periods of relatively good health interspersed with critical illness. The dynamic aspect of AIDS presents special research problems and has implications for care and prevention.

The similarities and differences between AIDS and other acute and chronic conditions and health care needs point to further issues. For example, caring for persons with AIDS raises several generic research questions about how informal social supports are mobilized in the care of family and friends—or how the current health care system responds to long-term care needs. In many ways the problems (such as accessibility, quality, coordination, and costs of care) faced by AIDS patients of all ages in the search for health care are very similar to those experienced by older persons who have traditionally sought long-term care.

However, the particular nature of the disease—its infectious, life-threatening, and stigmatizing character—also produces individual and societal responses that are unique to such diseases. We see, for example, that stigmatized conditions can affect an individual's recognition of illness symptoms, the ways in which others respond to persons with such stigmatized conditions, and the entire process of seeking and obtaining care.

Thus a deeper understanding of the similarities and differences in experiences with the epidemic is needed. The risk of infection and strategies for prevention of AIDS vary widely across geographic regions in the United States and elsewhere. To what extent can we generalize experiences from areas with high caseloads and active AIDS support groups to other areas where AIDS is relatively rare? National as well as cross-national comparisons are important for an understanding of transmission routes as well as of differences in personal and societal responses to the disease.

It has also been noted that AIDS is not a unitary phenomenon, but has different risk factors and consequences in different populations. Previous chapters have documented the various ways in which age defines the AIDS epidemic. The special vulnerabilities of the older population cannot be neglected (e.g., older people's relative lack of knowledge about AIDS and its major transmission routes, their increased susceptibility to AIDS conversion following exposure, the greater threats to their health based on age-related biological changes and existing co-morbidities, and their lack of resources for costly medical care).

Older persons are also seen as resources themselves in the fight against AIDS. If effective educational programs are disseminated to them, older persons cannot only modify their own risky behaviors but can also serve as change agents for influencing risk-taking behaviors and for advocating behavioral change (e.g., safe sex practices) to younger relatives. Middle-aged and older persons will also undoubtedly serve as frontline caregivers for family members with AIDS.

SETTING A RESEARCH AGENDA

While social and behavioral research in general has burgeoned in the last decades, specific knowledge about AIDS and aging is scanty. This volume has identified many research issues needing specific study. There are both short-term and long-term research agendas and methodologies. Some research projects could begin immediately and be completed in a relatively short time (e.g., analysis of existing survey data on older people's attitudes about AIDS and persons with AIDS). Research on psychosocial factors in the natural course of the disease, however, requires longitudinal follow-up throughout the latency and disease period. Other types of research questions (e.g., realistic forecasting of the demographic implications of AIDS for middle-aged and older persons) depend on the adaptation of existing forecasting models and a better understanding of underlying disease processes and the course of the disease. In all cases, a phasing of research is required, with accumulating knowledge from early studies stimulating future research directions.

Target Populations and Methodological Issues

There is a need to develop strategies for approaching the important research questions identified throughout this volume. In addition to specifying needed research questions, there are major considerations of the identification and recruitment of populations for study—especially when research questions focus on those who have been exposed to the HIV virus, who are seropositive, or who have manifest symptoms of AIDS or associated opportunistic infections.

At the same time that the importance of obtaining representative samples is emphasized, many problems in meeting this research ideal (due to the highly personalized and intimate nature of sex and AIDS research) have been identified. In addition to large-scale surveys, there is also a place for more intensive qualitative studies for specific research questions not readily adaptable to closed-ended survey questioning. Researchers need not be tied to any particular population or methodology—these should be guided by the particular research objectives that have been posed by the epidemic.

Several different target populations, often requiring special research strategies, can be identified:

1. Old people constitute *one segment of the general population* in surveys of knowledge and attitudes toward AIDS or persons with AIDS. Investigation of this segment entails either adding AIDS-related questions to general surveys or conducting AIDS-specific studies. Many research teams currently investigating AIDS do not include scientists with aging expertise or with an understanding of special issues in conducting research on older persons. It is strongly recommended that age-relevant methodological expertise be available when adding an aging component to any general population survey, since problems may arise in attempting to use the general protocols for older persons.

2. *Special subpopulations* are often of interest within the general population. For example: How do older persons needing or already in long-term care settings—and their families or other caretakers—react to AIDS or PWA?

3. Middle-aged or older persons as *caregivers for PWA* may need to be identified. Research studies can be directed both to informal and to paid caregivers. Study populations can often be located through PWA groups or organized groups of caregivers. However, researchers using this sampling approach must be alert to possible bias toward those with more serious conditions or toward areas where AIDS is more prevalent.

4. Particular *high-risk groups* within the older population must often be identified. Four major groups are already well known: older gay/bisexual males, IV drug abusers, persons who received early (before 1985) nonscreened blood transfusions, and those who engage in unprotected sex with members of high-risk groups. New high-risk groups may emerge in the future as HIV infection becomes prevalent in other populations or whenever presently undetected HIV infection turns into full-blown AIDS. It will be difficult to obtain representative samples of some high-risk groups (e.g., older bisexuals, who are often secretive about their sexual behaviors). Older persons who live in affluent retirement communities who may be engaging in unprotected sex with multiple partners illustrate one as yet unidentified population group for study.

5. For some research objectives, *older persons with AIDS-associated opportunistic infections or HIV infection* may need to be located. There are a range of social and behavioral research problems here. At present the numbers of older persons with AIDS or associated opportunistic infections are thought to be relatively small, and the problem of studying populations with rare events is well recognized. Research subjects may be hard to identify other than through health care settings, and this will predictively result in the inclusion of persons

in advanced stages of the disease rather than those at earlier stages. It is particularly difficult to identify older persons at early stages of HIV infection —especially those who do not even know they are infected. Various strategies for attempting to deal with this problem are suggested throughout the book. Yet the difficulties are great, and they are compounded by added problems of confidentiality and legal issues of disclosing information about PWA.

Substantive Issues

The National Institute on Aging (NIA) initially identified four broad research areas on AIDS and aging and requested assistance from outside advisors on what was known and needed to be known about the social and behavioral factors. The following represents our summary of important research questions in the original four areas as well as two additional areas identified during subsequent advisory discussions. Our summary is designed to illustrate unanswered research questions as currently identified by NIA and its advisors. The four initial identified areas were as follows:

1. *Sexual attitudes and practices.* It is quite clear that systematic information on older people's sexual attitudes and practices is lacking. In recognition of the need for population-based information in this area, a national survey is being planned at the time of this writing. Starting in 1988, NIA is working with the National Institute of Child Health and Human Development (NICHD) and other federal agencies to design such a survey and to pilot-test the special issues in interviewing older people about their sexual attitudes and behaviors. Numbers of AIDS cases are available (as "numerators"), but basic demographic information is missing on "denominators" (e.g., how many older people are engaging in sexual activities? What kinds of sexual activities? How often? With whom?). Such baseline information is needed in order to understand transmission routes and the potential spread of AIDS in the older population. In addition to counting numbers of sexual partners and sexual practices, the social and behavioral conditions under which particular sexual practices are developed or reinforced must be investigated.
2. *Impact of AIDS on older persons' health care attitudes and behaviors—and on the health care system itself.* While health services research in general has been slow to examine older persons' health attitudes and behaviors (as compared to those of younger persons), even less is known about the impact that AIDS has on such attitudes and behaviors of older persons or on their health care providers. Do fears of contagion or new health care protocols (e.g., gloves and masks) reduce older people's willingness in general to seek appropriate health care? What are health care professionals' fears about AIDS and their attitudes toward clients with AIDS? How do they treat older persons with

AIDS or older family members who are caring for AIDS patients? What modifications are required in the already overloaded existing health care structures and practices (home care, community services, nursing home care, or hospice care) to deal with rising numbers of persons with AIDS? How can these structures and practices be adapted and widely used to meet the long-term care needs of older persons?

3. *Impact of a diagnosis of AIDS on families and social networks.* Research suggests that many persons with AIDS rely on their parents for care in the final stages of the disease. Indeed, several studies have found that almost 50% of AIDS patients are living with their parents. There are, however, several general research questions on the mobilization of social and family supports. How do older persons respond as caregivers to younger persons with AIDS? What are older family members' reactions and coping responses when they learn that their adult children have AIDS, and when these "children" come back to live with them? What are the economic and employment implications of having to care for an adult child with AIDS? How do older family caregivers interface with younger friends of PWA? What social supports are available to older PWA who may not be part of highly visible and organized risk groups? How are formal and informal care services linked?

4. *Research on forecasting societal implications of the spread of AIDS.* This fourth area is critically important in preparing for the future—but it is currently hindered by the poor quality of existing epidemiological and behavioral data. (Note comments on sexual attitudes and practices in #1 above.)

There is a need to examine the feasibility of adapting current demographic and epidemiological forecasting models to the special situation of AIDS. Two complementary approaches are identified in this book: (1) the development of strategies for combining multiple local data sets to map the spread of AIDS geographically and (2) the combining of demographic and biosocial models to improve predictions of the transmission of and spread of AIDS through society. New forecasting models that utilize both approaches are needed.

Biosocially valid models must take into account the natural history of the disease process, including both the heterogeneity of individual vulnerabilities and the known risks of contracting AIDS. The research task of preparing such models is complex and demands attention to many areas. What is the possibility of a future rise in AIDS cases among older people because of the well-known declines with aging in the immune system? What might be the impact of AZT and other drug therapies on the survival of AIDS patients and thus of their frequencies in the population?

Improved forecasting models are also needed for assessing the impact of a potential spread of the AIDS epidemic on the age composition of the population. A sharp rise in AIDS-related mortality among younger persons could contribute to a more rapid "aging of the population," as seen in some African countries. More generally, we need to understand the impact of any accelerated spread of the epidemic on the family, the health care system, the workforce, and other social institutions. To suggest an extreme example, what would happen to care and support of older persons if substantial numbers of younger persons—the current caretakers—were to die prematurely?

The two additional research areas brought into focus during the subsequent advisory discussions relate to the course of the disease and prevention efforts.

5. The *natural history of the disease* and *the process of coping* along the illness continuum need study. Questions are raised about how biomedical and psychosocial factors interact to affect the onset and course of the disease, the functional loss associated with the progression of the disease, increasing co-morbidity as the disease progresses, and the changing long-term care and acute-care case mix at different stages of the disease. There has been some work, but more is needed, on the psychoneuroimmunology of the condition and how psychosocial factors such as depression or sense of personal control affect the natural history and progression of the disease. Important research issues on decision making at the end of life and research questions about the processes of death and dying are becoming increasingly imperious.

6. *Prevention and behavioral interventions.* While there has been an increase in the number and types of public health and educational campaigns to combat the AIDS epidemic, there has been little attention to how interventions need to be tailored to middle-aged and older populations. Two types of interventions are involved: (1) the reduction of high-risk behaviors associated with AIDS and (2) the provision of support to help older persons cope in their caregiving roles. Such questions arise, for example, as: How will information about AIDS (e.g., the 1988 household mailing by the U.S. Surgeon General) effect or fail to effect the desired changes in behavior among older persons as compared with younger persons? If interventions are initially successful, does compliant behavior persist among older persons?

CARE ISSUES

Health care research on the social and behavioral aspects of AIDS is another area in which older people are involved, not only as recipients of care but also as caregivers.

Older People's Relationship to Care

The various ways in which older persons are intricately linked to AIDS-related care are not widely recognized. There is, however, substantial evidence on several fronts. Older persons are: (1) care recipients (that 10% of new AIDS cases in the U.S. are 50 years old and older has been repeatedly reported throughout this volume); (2) informal care providers for spouses, children, and grandchildren (families consistently provide the bulk of long-term care, and, although same age peers might provide more care for PWA than other chronically ill persons, studies show that approximately 50% of PWA are living with and receiving care from their parents); (3) co-users of health care (at the time of writing, PWA and older persons are in different health care streams, but there is some overlap in acute-care and home health settings), and (4) paid providers of care (already some professional health care providers are themselves older people, and substantial numbers of nonprofessional middle-aged and older persons are being recruited for the growing home health and nursing home industry). While there are active support groups for PWA, there are relatively fewer groups that provide support for their caregivers (this is in contrast to very active support groups for caregivers of older people with Alzheimer's Disease).

Economic and Organizational Aspects of Care

The national cost of care for AIDS is already staggering (total direct costs for 1986 have been estimated at 1.64 billion dollars), and these costs are expected to increase as persons already infected develop AIDS, as new persons become infected, and as new treatments prolong life without reducing medical care problems. Efforts are under way to obtain more reliable estimates of total costs of AIDS care, to compare these costs to other diseases, and to evaluate the cost-effectiveness of various health care and social services.

Yet the concern with care for PWA and those experiencing related conditions is already immediate. Problems in obtaining and financing appropriate care are one indication of longstanding inadequacies in the American health care system that older persons have faced for some time. Although inadequacies of health care have been decried as a crisis for both PWA and older persons, as of 1989 few fundamental changes have been made in the existing health and social service systems, especially with respect to meeting long-term care needs. We speculate that the combined health care demands of these two populations may overwhelm the current system and actually become the driving force for encouraging needed changes in the organization, delivery and financing of health care.

Common Concerns of PWA and Older People

While persons with AIDS and older people without AIDS can be characterized by some as competitors for limited health care resources, the interdependence of different groups with common needs cannot be overlooked. A broader view may be taken that emphasizes the sharing of different coping strategies and models of care. We are already seeing, for example, the utilization of innovative models of care for PWA that broaden and modify long-term care models traditionally used by older persons with chronic illnesses and functional disabilities.

An evaluation of the best experiences with a variety of long-term care approaches for PWA can feed back into future modifications in long-term care for older persons. For example, the issue of whether integrated or segregated care units are best for subgroups of older people with particular diseases (e.g., special care units for persons with Alzheimer's Disease) is still an open question. An examination of the pros and cons of specially dedicated units for AIDS patients may shed additional light on this broader issue. Moreover, the introduction of "universal precautions" in response to the AIDS epidemic is undoubtedly having far-reaching benefits in reducing other infections and medical complications.

Similarities and differences in the effects of AIDS and aging on health care experiences are also of interest. The interface between informal and formal care is a major health care policy issue that is hotly debated in the current cost-containment atmosphere. Especially in the aging and health care arena, there are fears that the availability of formal services will reduce the family's willingness to care for their relatives. However, there is evidence to suggest that families continue to provide substantial amounts of care for older relatives even after the introduction of formal services, although it is not clear whether the same situation applies to those caring for PWA. It is still an open question whether the uniqueness of the medical and social aspects of AIDS necessitates a greater reliance on formal care than is required for the health conditions typically found in older persons.

Much research has noted the impact of a subtle ageism in older persons' search for health care and in health care providers' responses to older people. Similar concerns are raised about PWAs' definition of their illness and their treatment by care providers. The speculation is that the scientific and medical community's response is similarly influenced by ageism and by the stigma attributed to the special conditions of AIDS. This may help explain why care for both PWA and older persons has lagged behind other categories of persons needing care.

A Paradigm for Care

Our efforts to date call attention to the promising paradigm for examining the care of persons with AIDS that is outlined in the earlier chapter by Stall, Catania, and Pollack. This model calls for the study of differences in care (formal and informal) between two populations: persons with AIDS versus those with other life-threatening chronic conditions such as cancer. Within the AIDS population, two related research questions may be addressed by comparing subpopulations: (1) differences in care when AIDS is contracted through stigmatizing behavior (homosexual contact) and nonstigmatizing behavior (blood transfusion) and (2) differences in care for younger as compared to older AIDS patients. The implications of this model are worthy of further investigations.

PUBLIC EDUCATION AND PREVENTION

The accumulating scientific knowledge, as indicated in this volume, can be useful in the formation of public education and prevention strategies. The eventual transferability of scientific knowledge to public prevention efforts should be an explicit goal of research on social and behavioral aspects of AIDS. Identification of the most effective health promotion programs must be based on an understanding of the epidemiology of AIDS-related risk factors in persons of different ages and on surveys of AIDS-related public knowledge, attitudes, and behaviors.

Target Populations

The current state of the science suggests the potential effectiveness of several public health approaches and targets. At least four such targets are evident:

1. *General public information.* Education of the public at large is needed to reduce the public's unwarranted fears of AIDS and to eliminate subtle and overt discriminatory practices toward PWA. Programs should be designed to impart accurate and nonjudgmental information about AIDS. One emphasis might be to counter the stigma associated with AIDS and PWA by explicit messages that AIDS is not restricted to any one particular population group and that it occurs at all ages.
2. *General public education for older persons.* Social surveys on AIDS-related knowledge, attitudes, and behaviors suggest the need for specific education targeted at older persons: The general population of older persons knows less and is more misinformed about AIDS than the younger population. In addition to the general public education approach, there is a need to pay special attention to older persons by directing information to organizations affiliated with older persons (the American Association for Retired People now has a public statement on the prevention of AIDS), professionals working with older persons (e.g., doctors and religious counselors), and sites where older people congregate (e.g., retirement communities or senior centers).

3. *Education for populations with high-risk behaviors.* The epidemiological investigation of transmission sources among AIDS cases suggests several targets for interventions in groups at high risk. Contrary to popular assumptions about asexuality in old age, there is evidence that coital frequency in many older people is adequate for the transmission of the HIV virus, especially given the biological vulnerability associated with old age. Within the older population many are not aware of implications of their sexual behaviors for HIV transmission, or of the need for protective measures. Special attention should be paid to (1) persons who received pre-1985 blood transfusions, (2) gays and bisexuals, especially those who are not part of active gay communities, and (3) the sexual partners of these persons who may not be aware of their partners' infection. These are the populations currently identified at highest risk (IV drug abuse has been a less critical source of transmission among older than younger people). It is likely that the contribution of these special groups to the AIDS epidemic will lessen over time as public health campaigns are directed to them. In addition, we need to be aware of other target populations whose current high-risk status may be hidden (e.g., middle-aged and older women) and who may fuel future waves of the epidemic.

4. *Training of health care providers.* There is an inadequate supply of health care providers trained in care of AIDS patients—either as specialists or as general practitioners with knowledge of AIDS diagnosis, treatment, and management and with the psychosocial skills necessary for interacting with PWA and their families. Thus there is a pressing need for additional formal and on-the-job training of health care workers. This training, as our various advisors agreed, should not be restricted to high-level professionals such as doctors, dentists, and nurses but should include workers at all levels (such as health care attendants in nursing homes and home health aides). Given older persons' relative lack of AIDS-related knowledge, it is especially critical that persons working with older persons have a rudimentary knowledge of AIDS. There have already been reports of cases of long delays in the diagnosis of AIDS in older persons due to lack of recognition of presented symptoms.

Behavioral Change Strategies

Once the target populations are identified, a key principle underlying behavioral change strategies is the need to tailor the particular interventions to both the condition and the population being addressed. The heterogeneity of AIDS as a disease calls for designing different strategies for populations of different age and with different risk factor profiles. Thus, programs for younger persons might focus on reducing high-risk behaviors such as having sex with multiple partners. For postreproductive older people with exposure to the virus through blood transfusions, the main message might be to increase their awareness of the risks to both new and lifelong sexual partners and to encourage the use of protective measures during sexual intercourse.

The public health mandate to respond to the AIDS epidemic underscores how little we know about motivating and changing health behaviors in general—and it reflects the specific neglect of older persons in behavioral research. The problem is further compounded by the need to understand the special considerations imposed by the uniqueness of the social, behavioral, and medical aspects of AIDS. Yet we know the importance of the social and behavioral context for influencing health-related behaviors and maintaining recommended behavioral changes. This context requires special attention in research on sexual behaviors, which by nature are social phenomena and dependent on interactions with others.

Prevention models based on existing social and behavioral principles of behavior change are useful in designing interventions. Two models described in this volume are illustrative. The first describes the "illness career," which involves at-risk behaviors, becoming infected, developing AIDS, seeking health care, becoming terminally ill, and dying (see chapter by McKinlay et al.). The second risk reduction model specifies a conceptual framework for understanding the conditions that encourage or impede the processes of behavioral recognition, commitment, and action for reducing HIV risk behaviors (see chapter by Catania et al.). Such models are useful in designing strategies for primary and secondary public health interventions.

Contributions and Limitations of Public Health Interventions

The importance of public health interventions cannot be underestimated in this as in other epidemics. Even if a "silver bullet" were found tomorrow that prevented or cured AIDS, it would still be essential to understand the social and behavioral dimensions of AIDS transmission and prevention. It is clear that AIDS-related behaviors have been changed dramatically since the beginning of the epidemic, especially in the gay community, where education campaigns have been widely disseminated. Yet the dynamics of behavioral change for different age groups are imperfectly understood, and one critical unanswered question is the extent to which behavioral change strategies generally employed with younger persons can be useful with older persons as well. Clearly, further study is needed to clarify the complex interactions among aging, health, and behavioral processes.

THE AIDS EPIDEMIC AS A CATALYST

One benefit derived from the discussions of the AIDS epidemic in this book is that they force us to recognize the AIDS epidemic as a catalyst for thought and intervention. The discussions compel us to review previous thinking about many issues and policies, to confront new and unresolved ethical dilemmas, and indeed to recognize the epidemic as itself a source of numerous societal innovations.

Public Policies

The AIDS epidemic calls attention to the need to reexamine the delicate balance between civil liberties and public health policies. Public opinions on these issues are often informed more by fears of the epidemic than by scientific understanding of the development and spread of AIDS. Screening and testing, confidentiality versus mandatory reporting, protective control measures (e.g., quarantine), professional obligations, and individual rights to and decisions about treatment all are being widely debated. The outcomes will have direct implications for AIDS prevention, care, and research. For example, mandatory testing and reporting policies, coupled with discriminatory practices (in employment, housing, and insurance practices), may act only to discourage voluntary testing and the acceptance of appropriate public health measures. Although the specific legislative decisions and regulations may change over time, it is increasingly important to examine how such policies affect health care decisions and the quality of life for PWA and their caregivers.

Care Implications

AIDS also serves as a catalyst for addressing issues of terminal care and the right to die, which are major—but often avoided—concerns in health care for older persons. The AIDS crisis forces us to reexamine professional obligations and the interactions between health care providers and their clients. We have learned from experience with other health conditions (e.g., public health efforts to reduce cardiovascular disease) the importance of combining any screening and testing with education and counseling. Such lessons in helping health care professionals to provide more humane care for AIDS patients can be used to improve care for older persons as well.

Research Implications

Since issues of informed consent and confidentiality have turned out to be especially important in AIDS-related research, they are affecting the researchers' ability to obtain needed populations for study. Moreover, some high-risk persons and PWA are no longer interested in participating in descriptive clinical or epidemiological studies and are demanding access to treatment and programs as a condition of their participation. Further, the "research purity" of traditional clinical trials is being affected by subjects' refusal of nontreatment assignments or their unauthorized use of untested but promising treatments.

Innovations in Social Institutions

The AIDS epidemic is prompting new and sometimes innovative responses from the various social institutions that bind society together. Many implications for the health care industry have already been discussed here in some detail. In addition, the complex of educational, legal, family, work, financial, military, and other social institutions is affected by the epidemic in new ways, and their response will influence the future directions and social consequences of AIDS. In some cases these institutions appear to be mutually supportive in the actions undertaken; at other times AIDS-related institutional policies operate at cross purposes. For example, a goal of public health organizations is to encourage voluntary testing, whereas both insurance and employment regulations are causing some persons at risk to avoid testing altogether. Also involved is the entire world of entertainment, art, and fashion, which has been especially hard hit. Because all these institutions can be expected to experience disruption, even substantial chaos, in the future, new forms and structures are bound to take shape.

Exacerbation of Social Cleavages

An unfortunate outcome has been produced by the lack of a coherent AIDS policy, which inadvertently fueled the initial spread of the epidemic. A consensus has been building that this lack continues to exacerbate the underlying tensions left unanswered. The association of AIDS with disadvantaged or highly stigmatized groups (e.g., minorities, gay or bisexual males, drug abusers) has threatened to increase societal cleavages and to undo recent gains in civil rights. The tendency in 1988 toward judicial support of the basic rights of PWA and the strong federal directives against discriminatory policies in various social and medical domains are encouraging. Nevertheless, our reading of some of the international responses to AIDS suggests that the epidemic sometimes serves to reinforce existing xenophobic tendencies, as in some countries that restrict travel on the basis of AIDS.

Implications for Positive Innovations

On a more positive note, the AIDS epidemic has also generated new organizational structures and solidarities. There has been a strong mobilization of voluntary networks, and advocacy groups for the prevention and care of AIDS are becoming empowered and are providing the basis for new social movements. It is primarily in response to intensive lobbying by such AIDS advocacy groups that the availability of drugs approved by the Federal Drug Administration—a normally long and bureaucratically tedious procedure—has been accelerated.

AIDS AND AGING: A NEW FORM OF SYNERGY?

These "Notes for the Future" have pointed to a few of the many important research, prevention, care, and social issues involved in examination of AIDS in an aging society. We have seen that older persons—as either recipients, providers, or co-sharers of care—are inextricably implicated in the AIDS epidemic. A latent message from this volume is that AIDS and aging issues are so intertwined as to produce a new order of synergism.

On the one hand, the further study of social and behavioral aspects of AIDS in middle-aged and older populations will add to our understanding of the antecedents and consequences of the epidemic. Unquestionably, the strong and unprecedented multidisciplinary efforts by biomedical, social, and behavioral scientists of many persuasions will eventually uncover the natural history of AIDS, identify risk factors for its spread, and design programs and policies for containing and alleviating its social consequences.

On the other hand, highly focused study of AIDS will, in turn, feed back into our general knowledge of the health-related attitudes and behaviors of older persons and further illuminate their interactions with family and health care systems. A more detailed understanding of how social supports are mobilized for the care of persons with AIDS, together with innovative ways for organizing and delivering long-term care, will eventually benefit all older persons and their families.

The place of older persons in the AIDS epidemic can no longer be overlooked. Knowledge of the complex interactions of biomedical, behavioral, and social aging processes that influence risk factors and prevention strategies in the later years is rapidly being added to the scientific arsenal available to researchers, practitioners, and policy makers combating AIDS.

INDEX

DATE DUE

FEB 27 1991			
AP 15 '92			
NOV 09 1993			